Atkins Diet Beginners' Crash Course

Your Quick Start Plan for Simple, Fast, Effective Weight Loss and Better Health - Includes meal plan and recipes!

Robert M. Fleischer

Publishing

Atlanta, Georgia USA

ISBN 978-1-491284-15-5

9 781491 284155 >

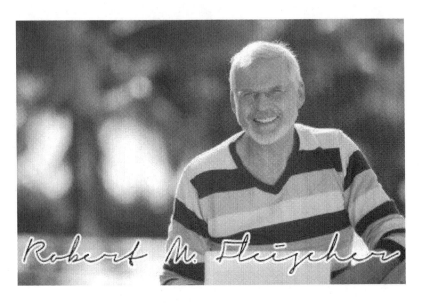

Copyright © 2012 Robert M. Fleischer

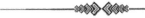

Readers' Feedback

"This worked when nothing else did."

★★★★★ Deborah Young – Connecticut

"I've lost inches from my waist and I feel totally alive! I can't recommend this book strongly enough. Thank you!"

★★★★★ Michael Carter – Boston

"Everything I needed in a nutshell. This guide really opened my eyes to how stress affected the size of my waistline."

★★★★★Jane Fortini - Rockhampton

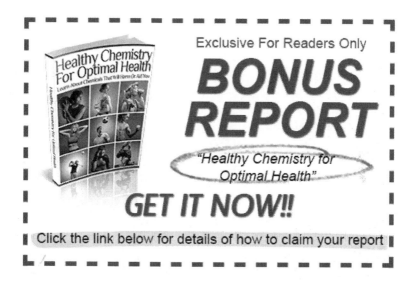

Exclusive Bonus Download: Healthy Chemistry for Optimal Health

Thousands Have Used Chemicals To Improve Their Medical Condition!

Is the fact that you would like to learn to use chemicals for your health but just don't know how and this is making your life difficult... maybe even miserable?

First, you are NOT alone! It may seem like it sometimes, but not knowing how to get better your skills is far more common than you'd think.

Your lack of knowledge in this area may not be your fault, but that doesn't mean that you shouldn't -- or can't -- do anything to find out everything you need to know to finally be a success!

So today -- in the next FEW MINUTES, in fact -- we're going to help you GET ON TRACK, and learn how you can quickly and easily get your skills under control... for GOOD!

With this product, and it's great information on chemicals it will walk you, each and every chemicals and it's use to help you get all the info you need to be health.

In This Book, You Will Learn:

- The Chemistry Of The Blood
- The Relationship Between The Biology And The Chemistry Of The Blood
- Dangerous Chemicals To The Body
- Good Chemicals To The Body
- 10 Reasons Why You Should Avoid The Bad Chemicals

And so much more!

<u>Download this guide and start improving your health NOW</u>

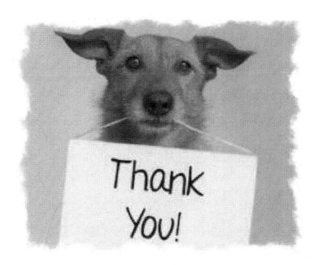

Thank you for downloading my book. Please REVIEW this book on Amazon. I need your feedback to make the next version better. Thank you so much!

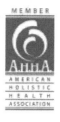

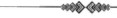

Books by Maggie Fitzgerald
The 7-Day Acid Reflux Diet
The 3-Step Diabetic Diet Plan
The Anti-Inflammatory Diet Plan
Ketogenic Diet Crash Course
Atkins Diet Beginners' Crash Course

www.amazon.com/author/robertfleischer

Is This Book for You

Times change, life changes, and people have to follow in their wake. And diets have to do the same. The Atkin's diet is not new, and yet it is. As time has gone by and people's eating habits moved in a different direction, it had to follow suit. So here's the new Atkin's diet.

I wrote this book because I truly believe that there is huge need for this book right now; obesity, like it or not, is one of the biggest epidemics of our era. There've never been so many obese people as there are today, not only in the western industrialist world, but also the eastern developing one. There are a lot of things to blame for this, but most of all we should blame ourselves and our unhealthy habits.

If you read this book you'll come to understand that where there's a will, there's indeed a way. If you follow my instructions to the letter, if you eat the right things and exercise regularly soon enough you'll see the pounds slipping away from your body, leaving it healthier and stronger, in a better shape that it has ever been. Now is not the time of talking but doing; follow the diet, reap the rewards.

TABLE OF CONTENTS

Disclaimer

While all attempts have been made to provide effective, verifiable information in this Book, neither the Author nor Publisher assumes any responsibility for errors, inaccuracies, or omissions. Any slights of people or organizations are unintentional.

This Book is not a source of medical information, and it should not be regarded as such. This publication is designed to provide accurate and authoritative information in regard to the subject matter covered. It is sold with the understanding that the publisher is not engaged in rendering a medical service. As with any medical advice, the reader is strongly encouraged to seek professional medical advice before taking action.

Author's Introduction

No matter where you live, how much money you make, how many kids you have, or how old you are, it's possible that you struggle with your weight. People who are extremely successful, people who used to be college athletes, and people who are very motivated can all be overweight; it's a condition that crosses racial, economic, social, familial, and political boundaries, and it's something that's getting a lot worse. According to some estimates, as many as 70% of people in the United States are classified as overweight or obese. And why is this the case? Because gaining weight is easy, and losing weight is hard. Or that's what we tell ourselves. And, in fact, that's true, if you've been on the modern, Western diet your entire life, like almost everyone else in the country. But many people have been finding out over the past few decades that losing weight doesn't have to be so hard. In fact, it can be easy, satisfying, and sustainable, without constant calorie-counting, excessive exercise, or a huge amount of self-denial. This is the secret of the low-carbohydrate diet.

Low-carb diets, especially the Atkins Nutritional Approach, have received a lot of criticism over the past few decades. And, to be honest, some of it was very accurate. But there's a lot of sensationalism out there, and the diet itself has changed, and it has become one of the best and most effective ways to lose weight that you can choose. If done correctly, it's relatively easy, extremely effective, safe, and sustainable, which is something that not very many diets can say. I've tried to lose weight on several occasions myself, and I can tell you: if you're not making changes to how your body uses calories, you're setting yourself up for failure. And changing how your body functions is the core principle of the Atkins diet. But we'll get to that a bit later.

11

There is a huge need for this book right now, as the weight of the average American slowly but steadily creeps upward. Healthcare costs are going up, group insurance provided by employers can be more difficult to come by, and we just don't have time to be unhealthy! It may sound like I'm overstating the dangers and difficulties of being overweight, but take my word for it: we are paying a huge cost every day, and we think that we can't do anything about it. But spend a month on the Atkins diet, and you'll discover, as I have, that this is just not true. You *can* get rid of that unsightly abdominal fat; you *can*have a beach-ready body; and you *can* reach a weight that makes you happy. It's time to stop listening to the mainstream media, the fad diet books, and the "experts" who say that you need to religiously measure every calorie that you eat. There's a better way, and this is it.

I sincerely hope that you enjoy this book as much as I enjoyed writing it, and I wish you the best of luck with your weight loss endeavors. I'm placing a valuable tool in your hands—don't be afraid to use it!

Sincerely,

Robert M. Fleischer

What You'll Get from This Book

Every diet has promises for you—they'll tell you that'll get a super model's body, or that you'll drop three dress sizes, or that you'll be the weight that you were in college, and sometimes they deliver. You start the diet, the pounds melt away, and you start heading toward your goals . . . but then you stagnate. You plateau in your weight loss, and you get frustrated. You might start gaining some of that weight back soon after losing it. You might start finding that the diet is much harder to maintain in the long-term than you thought it would be. And, eventually, you quit the diet because it's just too much work for such a small payoff. Sound familiar?

If this has happened to you, like it has to hundreds of thousands of other dieters, don't blame yourself! It's easy to get down on yourself when a diet just doesn't seem to work—it's easy to feel like you didn't put in enough work, or that if you had just a little more motivation, you'd succeed. But this isn't always true. In fact, I'd be willing to bet that *most* of the time, the fault actually lies with the diet itself.

Because most diets—especially the popular fad diets of the last couple decades—only ask you to change your habits. And while losing weight this way is possible, it's very difficult. But this diet is different; yes, it asks you to do some things differently. But it also changes the physiological processes in your body, turning it into a fat-burning machine. Don't worry—you don't need to understand the complex biochemistry behind these changes. All you have to do is follow the instructions that I lay out here for you and watch your fat start melting away!

The diet presented here has a lot of benefits. Foremost among them is that it actually works! It's effective, it's not hard, and it lets you work *with* your body instead of against it. In so many other diets, you'll feel like you're fighting against yourself to lose weight, and that's because you are. That's not what we're doing here. This diet helps train your body to turn stored fat into energy, helping you lose weight in a sustainable manner that won't leave you hungry, tired, and irritable all the time.

How will this diet do this? How can an Atkins diet, which has faced some serious criticism over the past few years, help you lose weight, cut belly fat, and improve your overall health in the process? The secret lies in the changes your body makes when you start a low-carbohydrate diet. As I mentioned a moment ago, there's some very complicated science behind this, but I've written this book specifically so you don't have to have a PhD in biochemistry to understand it. By cutting down on carbohydrates and selecting high-quality sources of protein and fat, you'll reduce the number of calories that you're consuming, increase the number of calories that you're burning, and train your body to use fat as a source of energy. This is the perfect equation for weight loss.

In the following sections, you'll learn the truth about carbohydrates, body fat, and how they're related. Ever wonder why you can eat a big breakfast and still end up hungry in two hours? You'll find out. After that, we'll discuss how the Atkins diet uses a low-carbohydrate diet to counteract the problems caused by carbohydrates.

I'll also be detailing how this revised version of the Atkins diet is both healthier and more effective than the traditional Atkins diet that has received so much criticism recently. Next, I'll be outlining the diet plan itself—telling you what, when, and how much to eat to optimize your fat burning potential in 21 days. And finally, I'll provide you with 21 recipes that will help you get started on the diet. By now, I'm sure you're anxious to get started. Let's go!

1. The Truth about Belly Fat

The focus of this diet is getting rid of fat. Specifically, belly fat. Why are we working so hard to get rid of belly fat? It seems like a simple question, but there are actually quite a few answers that you might hear. Let's take a look at a few of them one at a time.

1. Personal aesthetics.

Obviously, this is a big one. People want to slim down, especially around their waistlines, because they want to look trimmer, healthier, and more attractive. Everyone has their own definition of what's attractive, but this is a pretty common aspect. The modern Western society places a lot of value—far too much value, in fact—on being skinny. I'm going to go off on a bit of detour here, but it's important. I want to make sure to point out that slimming down is not the only thing that you can do to make yourself feel (and appear) more attractive; in fact, it's not even the most important thing.

By far, the most attractive attribute that any person can have, whether they're male or female, young or old, is a sense of confidence and self-worth. I know you've heard that before, but I feel very strongly about this, and I want to make sure that you don't misinterpret the purpose of this book. Yes, a flat stomach is attractive. But many people go too far in their pursuit of it.

All I'm saying here is that burning off a lot of fat is not worth killing yourself over. It's more important to have a healthy lifestyle, to know that you can be attractive no matter what the scale says, and that your figure does not define the quality of your person. That said, a balanced approach to looking better in a little black dress includes increased fitness, improved overall health, and weight loss. And a big part of effective weight loss is getting rid of excess fat from your body, especially from around your mid-section.

2. Improving overall health.

This is actually related both to the previous point and the next one. In the past few decades, there's been an increased emphasis on the value of being healthy. What exactly is meant by being "healthy" very much depends on who's saying it, but there are few, if any, people who would argue that improving your overall health is a bad thing. Some people want to be more fit, and set goals to exercise more. Others make efforts to improve their diet. And there are certainly people out there who want to just improve the functioning of their body in general. All of these are parts of improving your overall health, and cutting down the fat around your middle is really important in all of these things. If you want to get more fit by running, losing excess fat will help you by decreasing the amount of weight that you're moving with each step. If you're out to improve your diet without many other specific goals, you'll likely start losing fat because of it. And if you want to improve the functioning of your body, then losing fat is a fantastic way to go!

There are all kinds of ways that belly fat can mess with your body (keep reading to find out more about this). There are a lot of different facets of being healthy and living a healthy lifestyle, but they're all connected, and one of the points of connection is the loss of abdominal fat. So by setting this as a goal, you'll be setting yourself up for success when it comes to the more specific goals that you may have set in other areas.

3. Reducing risk of disease.

As we gain more insight into the causes and results of various diseases, it's become more clear that fat in the abdomen is not only unsightly, but also very unhealthy. It's been linked to a number of diseases, including some very serious ones like liver diseases, coronary heart disease, type-2 diabetes, insulin resistance, metabolic syndrome, stroke, and even dementia! It also increases the amount of inflammation in the body, and inflammation has been linked to another set of conditions that includes things like allergies and celiac disease (I'll provide a little more detail on why belly fat is so dangerous in the next section).

Obviously, belly fat is a more serious issue than just one that keeps you from wearing a bikini at the beach. In addition to improving your current health, getting rid of fat around your middle will help you stay healthier long into the future by reducing your risk of a number of diseases. And with the economy the way it is today, reducing the risk of disease can be not just a lifesaver, but a financial boon as well.

As jobs remain scarce, insurance prices continue to rise, and group insurance plans become shakier, it's going to get very costly to be overweight in the near future. Insurance companies ask you a lot of questions about various parts of your health, and being overweight or obese can significantly increase your risk in their eyes, meaning higher premiums or possibly even denials based on currently existing conditions. (I'm speaking from experience when I tell you that getting denied because of a condition that you have, even though it's been well-controlled for years, is extremely frustrating, and not something you want to deal with.) Even with the possibility of widely available government-funded healthcare on the horizon, it's not worth risking your financial future!

Of course, there are as many reasons for wanting to lose fat as there are people on diets (which is, to make a huge understatement, a lot). But many people don't realize just how *important* it is to reduce the amount of fat that you're carrying around.

1.1. The dangers of abdominal fat

I mentioned before that abdominal fat has a lot of negative health effects, but I didn't provide many details. For you to really understand why getting rid of this kind of fat is so crucial, I think it's important to understand exactly why it's so dangerous. First, I'll discuss an important distinction that many people don't even know exists: the two different kinds of belly fat. While you may think that it's all the same, there are actually some pretty big differences between the two different types.

The first type is called subcutaneous fat, and it's found right beneath your skin. Most of the fat in your body falls into this category: it's the fat that's most visible, and it's the kind that you can pinch with your fingers. While you might think that because there's so much *more* subcutaneous fat in the body, it's the more dangerous kind, but you'd be wrong there. The more dangerous kind is called visceral fat, and is stored exclusively in the abdomen. It's actually stored behind your abdominal muscles, in the abdominal cavity, where your organs are. Visceral fat has a number of negative effects, including

disruption of hormone function;

promotion of insulin resistance;

creation of chronic inflammation;

poor blood cholesterol levels;

increased risk of diabetes, high blood pressure, certain types of cancer, and atherosclerosis.

Obviously, all of these are very bad things, and should be avoided at all costs! If you know much about health, you'll see that a lot of these things are connected. Insulin and cortisol are hormones, and disruption of their normal function is linked to increased abdominal fat. High-carbohydrate diets which place a lot of stress on insulin and blood sugar management may cause high levels of inflammation, which is linked to a number of the other diseases. That's why it's so important that you treat your body as a holistic system and not just address a single symptom—if you only address your cholesterol levels, such as with cholesterol-lowering medications, for example, you won't know or treat the underlying cause, which may be causing more significant problems as well.

This is one of the reasons why so many diets that you may have tried in the past often fail—they, like a lot of Western medicine, only address a single factor in the equation. However, in the diet you'll read about in this book, you're not only addressing the symptoms, but you're also adjusting how the processes in your body work, and this is why it's so effective, as well as sustainable. If you only address one factor, and the treatment stops working, it's very difficult to continue with that treatment or to stay motivated to continue to work hard at it. But by addressing the body as a whole system, it's easier to keep your weight loss and general health management going in the right direction.

2. Atkins Diet Basics

What do you think of when you hear the phrase "Atkins diet"? Maybe you think of eating steak and eggs for breakfast. Or maybe you think of giving up fruit. And it's certainly possible that what comes to mind immediately is all of the controversy and argument over the diet over the past decade or so. No matter what you think of, it's likely that you have some misconceptions about the Atkins diet—and that's not at all your fault.

The principles behind the Atkins diet are scientifically sound, safe, and effective, but the way in which these principles were transformed into a popular diet plan weren't always very good. A lot of people associate low-carbohydrate diets with severe and negative effects on health; and while this is a great oversimplification, they do have some evidence to back up their claims. This chapter is here to help you get to know low-carbohydrate diets, why they work, and what went wrong with the first version of the Atkins diet (partly because your friends and family are almost certainly going to ask you if you're crazy when they find out you're on a low-carbohydrate diet).

2.1. The Atkins diet, version 1

Many people think that low-carb diets were invented in the 1960s or 1970s, when the Atkins diet first hit the scene. Others say that it was earlier, sometime in the 1920s, when low-carb diets were used to treat patients with epilepsy at the Mayo Clinic in Minnesota. Both of these are good guesses, but both are incorrect. Low-carbohydrate diets have actually been around since at least 400 b.c.— that's over two thousand years ago! And if this kind of diet has stuck around that long, it seems like it has to have some serious merits. Of course, what has counted as low-carbohydrate, the purpose of the diet, and exactly which foods were allowed have changed a lot, and continue to change on occasion. However, it's good to remember that low-carb diets haven't just been around for 40 or 50 years; they've been used for a very long time, and with a great deal of success.

The first version of the Atkins diet, however, had a few problems, and this is why low-carbohydrate diets have faced such criticism over the past several years. The diet was based on sound principles, and focused on turning the body from a carbohydrate-storing system into a fat-burning machine. Unfortunately, Dr. Atkins wasn't quite as clear as he could have been on a few points.

First of all, in early versions of the diet, he told dieters that they could eat as much meat and cheese as they wanted to, and still lose weight. If you know anything about how calories work, you'll see immediately that this is not a good idea (if you don't know much about calories, you'll learn in the next section). Even if the body is burning a huge amount of fat, you can't be consuming an unlimited amount and expect to lose weight (or stay healthy, for that matter).

Second, there was a big misunderstanding about how the diet progresses. As you'll see in the next chapter, there are several different phases of the diet, each with different requirements and restrictions. A lot of people thought that they had to just stick to the first phase, which has the most restrictions on carbohydrates. Keeping your carb intake that low for an extended period of time isn't a great idea, and if you follow the plan correctly, you'll slowly increase your intake of carbohydrates to get back up to a level that allows you to get the nutrients that you need.

And finally, it wasn't always made clear that the sources of fats and proteins that you consume on the diet are important. While the distinction between "good" fats and "bad" fats has been shown to be more complicated than many experts previously believed, there are still grades of quality when it comes to fats, and it's important to be getting the high-quality ones that your body can use effectively.

Because of all of these miscommunications and misconceptions, the first version of the Atkins diet was branded as being unhealthy and dangerous. However, a newer version of the Atkins diet has started to become more popular, and this "New Atkins," as some people call it, is what this book will focus on. After outlining the basics of a low-carbohydrate diet, I'll show you how to combine the revised version of the Atkins diet with exercise and stress management to help your body learn to turn fat into energy, and to use this to fuel steady, safe, and sustainable weight loss.

Unfortunately, most people don't realize that scientists have taken what Dr. Atkins started and refined it, turning it into a safe and viable diet. There's a lot of sensationalism out there regarding low-carbohydrate diets, and I urge you to read the next few sections so that you understand where these misconceptions came from and can help me show dieters and health gurus everywhere that the Atkins diet isn't just an excuse to eat all of the meat and dairy products that you want.

2.2. Why low-carb diets work

If you know someone who's tried a low-carb diet, you probably know that, when it comes down to it, they work. Especially during the first few weeks of the diet, you are likely to be surprised at how quickly you drop the first several pounds. Granted, a lot of the weight that you lose early on in any diet is water weight, and can come back pretty quickly, but even beyond this, the Atkins diet is very effective. There are some very complicated underlying biochemical reasons for this, but I'll skip the advanced physiology. In this section, you'll learn about the basic concepts that are behind the success of the Atkins diet, but don't worry; I don't have a PhD in physiology, and you don't need one either—I'll keep it as simple as possible.

1. Fueling the body.

All of your muscles and organs need fuel to work properly. Your muscles need fuel to contract, allowing you to move; your stomach needs fuel to digest foods and help get nutrients to the rest of your body; your brain needs fuel to think and manage the functions of all your organs. And this fuel is provided by calories, which can be derived from food or from stores in the body. Carbohydrates, fat, and protein in foods can be turned into energy during the digestion process, and both carbohydrates and fats are stored in the body to be used later.

Fat is a much more efficient energy source, as it provides 9 calories per gram, while carbohydrates and protein provide 4 calories per gram. In fact, so much energy can be derived from fat that if your body was able to break down all of its stored fat for use as energy, you'd be able to go for days and days without eating anything and you'd still be properly fueled. Unfortunately, because of the diet that has become so common in the modern Western world, the body is not very good at using stored fat for fuel. The aim of low-carbohydrate diets is fix this problem, and teach the body to use stored fat as an energy source.

There is a fourth source of energy, and it's actually quite important in the body's transition from being carbohydrate-dependent to being fat-fueled, but a full explanation would be quite complicated, so I'll only mention it briefly here. Ketones are a class of chemicals that are released by the liver when fat is broken down, and can be used by the body as a source of calories. The body is in a state of "ketosis" when there are a lot of ketones in the blood, and when this happens, it becomes less dependent on carbohydrate. When you're in ketosis, your body starts converting stored fat to energy. You might hear about ketogenic diets, or have people ask you about ketones or ketosis, so it's important to know that these words are all related to the low-carbohydrate diet and how it affects the body. If you'd like to learn more about ketosis and how the role that it plays in this diet, there are plenty of free resources online that will give you a detailed overview.

2. The body's response to carbohydrate restriction.

Carbohydrates, because they are easily obtained and stored, are a preferred source of energy—and while this may sound like a good thing, it often backfires. Our ancestors evolved to be very good at storing calories so that they could survive through times of food shortage. During long winters, droughts, or famines, people would rely on the calories they had stored in their bodies to fuel them while they couldn't find food, and these stores would get them through to the spring, or past the end of the famine.

However, this isn't really a necessary adaptation anymore—even when your city experiences a record-breaking winter, you can still just drive down to the corner grocery store. Our bodies haven't adapted to this comparative abundance yet, and still store all the extra calories that they can, which leads to weight gain unless you very carefully watch your calories; most of these stored calories come from carbohydrates, because they're easy to store.

So what happens when we drastically reduce the number of carbohydrates in our diet? The body starts looking for other fuels: first, it uses ketones, and then it uses fat. And as it uses these fuels, it becomes better and better at using them, so that even when carbohydrates become more available, it will still use the body's stores of fat as a fuel. This is the core concept behind the Atkins diet.

3. Hormones.

You may be surprised to discover that you've heard about a lot more hormones than you think you have: if you've heard of serotonin, melanin, dopamine, insulin, thyroxine, cortisol, or glucagon, you've heard about hormones. These are chemical substances that are used by the body to send messages. For example, when your metabolism needs to kick into high gear, your brain sends signals to your thyroid, and your thyroid sends signals to the rest of your body, through hormones. There are two hormones that are of interest to us here: insulin and cortisol.

Insulin is a hormone that is very closely related to glucose, a sugar that is found in carbohydrates. When sugar enters the blood, the level of insulin rises, and those carbohydrates are used or stored. In short, when insulin levels are high, more calories are stored in the body. By decreasing the number of carbohydrates that you consume, you'll keep your insulin levels low, which is crucial for the success of this diet and your weight loss plan. It also ensures, when insulin *is* released, that you respond correctly to it. If you constantly have a large amount of insulin in your body, you can start to develop resistance to its effects, which results in hyperglycemia (too much sugar in the blood), and this is a hallmark of diabetes. Not good. This is one of the areas in which the Atkins diet really helps your overall health and reduces your risk of diseases.

Cortisol is a hormone that's often linked with stress. When you experience mental or physical stress, cortisol is released—and while this is a good thing in the short-term, long-term exposure to it can have dire consequences, including the storage of more visceral fat. You may remember from our discussion of the two different types of abdominal fat that this is the more dangerous type. Cortisol is also related to inflammation, which, again, is good in the short-term, but has negative effects if it's persistent. As you'll find out in the next chapter, this diet prevents the buildup of cortisol in the body, thereby preventing the storage of belly fat.

Now that you understand these three factors, you have a pretty good idea of how this diet works. Keep these in mind throughout the next chapter so that you remember why each of the steps that I've listed there is important. It's definitely easier to motivate yourself to stick to the diet when you understand the purpose of each action!

2.3. Learning about carbohydrates

Okay, so it's becoming clear that significantly reducing your carbohydrate intake will result in healthy, sustainable weight loss. But before I go on, I want to make sure to point out that carbohydrates are not, in themselves, bad. In fact, they're quite necessary, as some organs can only function when they're fueled by carbohydrates. But not all carbs have the same effect on your body. So I'm going to use this section to give you an explanation of the different kinds of carbohydrates and how they affect your body.

1. Simple carbohydrates.

If there's one kind of carbohydrate that can be labelled as generally not helpful for losing weight, it's this category. Simple carbohydrates raise your blood sugar quickly, requiring a release of insulin (which can be bad for the reasons we discussed in the previous section). They also generally don't keep your full very long, making you hungry sooner, at which time you'll likely eat even more carbohydrates, prolonging the cycle (which is why you can eat a big breakfast of pancakes, and a muffin and still be hungry within a couple hours). This is one of the reasons why it's so difficult to lose weight for many people—they get addicted to sugars, and when they eat those sugars they re-enter the glucose / insulin cycle, causing the storage of a lot of fat. This is what we're trying to avoid. Simple carbohydrates are found in things like table sugar, candies, pre-processed and pre-packaged foods, and soda.

2. Complex carbohydrates.

On the other side of the spectrum, there are complex carbohydrates, which are of much higher quality and have more benefits. They don't raise your blood sugar as quickly, meaning you'll have a more steady level of energy after consuming them, and they're often found in foods that have more nutrients than foods with more simple carbs, so you get a double benefit there. Once you start restricting your carbohydrate intake, you'll want to aim to consume as many of your allowed grams of carbs from these sources as possible. Once you get past the first phase and are able to start consuming more, you should still be trying to eat only complex carbohydrates, but a few simple ones won't kill you. Complex carbohydrates are found in fruits and vegetables, whole grains, nuts and dairy products.

3. Fiber.

Unlike the previous two types of carbohydrate, fiber cannot actually be processed by the body, meaning it just passes through your digestive system without being absorbed. You might think that for this reason, it's not important, but it's actually very crucial both in weight loss and in maintaining your overall health. Fiber slows down the digestion of all of the foods in your stomach, meaning that no matter what you're eating, it'll give you a steadier blood sugar increase, reducing the chances of a big insulin spike.

It's also very important for your digestive health—because it can't be digested, it moves through your stomach, large intestine, and small intestine, picking up harmful substances along the way and helping your body remove them. Increased fiber intake is linked with a decreased likelihood of colon cancer, so this is something that you don't want to skip out on! Fiber is found primarily in whole grains.

The last thing I'll quickly discuss here is the glycemic index. You may be wondering how to tell if a source of carbohydrates is a simple or complex one, and whether there are degrees of blood sugar rise. The glycemic index (GI) is the answer to both of these questions. Every food has a GI value assigned to it that measures how quickly your blood sugar rises after eating it. On most scales, pure glucose is marked with 100, and all other foods are lower than this. So, foods high on the scale result in a rapid increase in blood sugar, which requires a rapid increase in insulin. Foods low on the scale, on the other hand, cause a steadier rise in blood sugar and a less drastic insulin response. For this reason, consuming low-GI carbs is preferable to high-GI ones. Here's a small list of foods with glycemic index values for each one:

Rice cakes: 82

Coca-Cola: 63

Banana: 62

All-Bran: 55

Yam: 54

Pear: 38

Skim milk: 32

Fettuccini: 32

Wheat tortilla: 30

Peanuts: 7

As you can see, the foods at the bottom of the list have some things in common. First, they're high in fiber. As I mentioned before, fiber slows down digestion and the subsequent blood sugar rise. Second, many of them are also high in protein or fat, both of which have an effect that is similar to fiber. When you're choosing carbohydrates, it's important to choose ones that are low on the scale as often as possible. You can find many long lists of foods and their associated GI values online.

Carbohydrates aren't the only foods with GI values, however. Every food raises your blood sugar to some degree, so every food has a value. This means that every meal that you consume has an overall GI value, and you should be seeking to keep that number low whenever possible. Because low-GI foods lower the GI value of all of the foods that are consumed at the same time, adding things like yogurt, cheese, or pumpernickel bread to your meal will reduce the overall effect on your blood sugar.

3. The Belly Fat Shred Diet

Throughout the first part of this book, we've gone over what you can expect from this diet, some facts about abdominal fat, the basics of the Atkins diet, and some key concepts related to carbohydrates. You're probably anxious to get started on the diet, so we'll now go over all of the steps you'll need to get form wherever you are right now to your goal weight. This chapter is divided into five sections, each of which is important. In the next chapter, you'll find two useful resources: a quick-start guide that contains the main principles of the diet, and a list of foods that are allowed or disallowed in certain phases of the diet. You can make a copy of these and keep them in your kitchen, or distribute them to friends, or do whatever you'd like with them—they're there as a useful tool for you to use in whatever way will help you reach your weight loss goals!

3.1. Goals and results

Before getting into the practical information you'll need to go on the Atkins diet to start getting rid of your abdominal fat, it's important to understand the process of setting and monitoring goals. Your progression through the four stages of the Atkins diet often depends on how close you are to your goal weight, so setting a weight that you're aiming for is a step that can't be overlooked. There are a few different ways to establish your goal, and which you use depends on largely on which one appeals to you most. All of these strategies are viable, so choose the one that you think will work the best for you!

1. The Atkins method.

In *Dr. Atkins' New Diet Revolution*, Robert Atkins recommends a very personal, qualitative method of determining your goal. Essentially, he asks you to think about the last time that you felt good about your weight, the weight at which you felt and looked your best, and suggests using this as your goal weight. Many people have a pretty specific number in mind when they think about this, and using it as a goal works very well for them.

Some people aim a bit higher than this, as getting back down to a weight that you haven't been at in decades might seem a bit too difficult. As you get older, you tend to gain some weight, and it gets harder to lose weight, so aiming for the weight that you were in high school might not be realistic. By combining the weight at which you looked and felt best with a bit of realism, you can come up with a good goal that will guide your weight loss efforts.

2. Ask a professional.

If you don't feel confident enough in your memory of your weight fluctuations, you can seek a more informed opinion. A physician is a good bet—they can take many factors into account and tell you the weight that you should be seeking to attain. You can certainly trust their opinion, as it's their job to know things like this. Many of them might not approve of the way that you're going to reach that goal weight, but they should be happy to help you decide what it is. Personal trainers are also good people to ask about weight loss, as they spend several hours every day coaching people to help them reach their goals, whether they're related to weight loss or fitness. Although they don't quite have the qualifications of a physician, they do have a lot of experience and can give you a good number to aim for.

3. Use the BMI chart.

Body mass index (BMI) is a measurement that's been in use for quite a while to see where people fall along the underweight-normal-overweight-obese spectrum. You can either use a formula (listed below) or a table (also below) to determine your current BMI as well as your goal BMI. The "normal" range is between 18.5 and 25, so choosing a goal within this range should be a safe bet. I put the word "normal" in quotes in the previous sentence because body mass index measurements can't take a lot of things into account; two people of the same height might have very different body types and therefore have different ideal weights. With that said, using the BMI scale is generally a pretty safe way to both take stock of your current situation and establish a reasonable goal to aim for.

$$BMI = ((\text{weight in lbs.}) / (\text{height in in.})2) \times 703$$

#mage1.jpg#

Whichever method you use to set a goal, it's a good idea to establish one before you get started on your diet. I know that it can be slightly disheartening to see that your goal is 40 or 60 or 80 pounds away, but it's a good idea to help keep you focused and to measure your progress. As this is a belly-fat-reducing diet, you can also set a waist measurement goal in addition to a weight goal. I don't have much guidance to offer on this, as it's a very personal measurement and only you have a good idea about where you should be aiming. Also, remember that you can lose quite a bit of weight without having a big change in your waist size, so be patient with this one. Think of it as a secondary goal.

Now that you have a goal, it's time to discuss ways of monitoring your progress toward that goal. Seeing your progress can be a very motivating thing, and I encourage you to keep a close eye on how your weight loss efforts are progressing. It can also be a good way to see which strategies are working and which aren't quite as effective, and it's important for determining when you progress through the different stages of the Atkins diet. Everyone has different ideas about monitoring, and different things work for different people, but I have a few recommendations that I'll share with you here.

1. Weigh in often.

Some people suggest weighing in once a week, while others recommend once every day . . . as I've said several times throughout this book, this is something that depends a lot on you. However, I think that the best way to go is to weigh in twice a week: Tuesday and Saturday. I think that weighing in every day encourages you to fixate too much on your weight, but that weighing in once a week isn't quite motivating enough. Two to three times seems to work best for me, so I generally recommend it. I find that I can keep pretty good track of my progress without becoming too fixated on my weight. But if weighing in once a month keeps you the most motivated, or you feel best when you weigh in twice a day, go for it. Just make sure you have a good idea of where you are.

2. Write down your goal and chart your progress.

One thing that many people (including myself) have been guilty of is changing their goals to better suit their progress. It's a natural thing to do—we want to feel like we're being successful in our endeavors, so we make it look like we are, no matter how it's going. The best way to keep yourself from doing this is to write your goal down and put it somewhere that it's very visible. Remind yourself of it on a regular basis so that you always keep it in mind. Stick a Post-It note on your computer or bathroom mirror, or change the desktop background of your phone to a picture that includes the number. Just do something so you see it very often. On a related note, write down your progress as well—write your weight on the calendar every time you weigh in, or make a thermometer chart—do whatever you need to do so that you don't forget how far you've come! It can be easy to get down on yourself if you've only lost a pound in the past three weeks. But it can help to remember that you've lost five, or ten, or twenty pounds before that!

3. Share your goal with people who will keep you accountable.

This is something that not everyone feels comfortable doing, but I strongly encourage it, no matter what. If you're the only person who knows your goal (or even that you're trying to slim down a bit), it's way too easy to adjust your goal, as there's no one to hold you accountable to it. You don't necessarily need someone who will harp on you until you get to your goal weight (unless that's what you want), but if you know that someone is going to ask you once a week, or once a month, if you've been getting closer to your goal, you're a lot more likely to keep making progress. Your spouse, or your kids, or your sibling, or a good friend or co-worker are all good bets. It can be even more motivating if the person who's holding you accountable is also trying to lose weight, as you can both help each other out. Trying to find a weight-loss partner is one of the most important pieces of advice that I can offer you!

3.2. 21 days to becoming a fat-burning machine

Success on the Atkins diet requires a long-term commitment, but I understand that you want to get up and running as fast as possible. Fortunately for you, I've condensed a lot of the important parts of the diet into a 21-day plan that will kickstart your weight loss and help you shed the first several pounds and inches from your belly. After detailing this three-week plan, I'll give you tips on how to progress with the diet to keep the weight coming off.

During these first weeks, you can expect a number of things, some of which are positive and some less so. On the positive side, you'll likely see your weight drop a few pounds. This is due to a number of factors, including reduced caloric intake, reduced water weight, and increased calorie burning through exercise.

Exactly how much you'll lose depends on your body type and how overweight you are to begin with, but it's reasonable to expect five pounds or so within the first three weeks. Several people on the forums at lowcarbfriends.com have shared their success stories, and quite a few have lost 15 or even 20 pounds in a month! However, because you're making significant changes to your diet, you may also experience cravings, withdrawal-like symptoms (which should tell you that this is a great thing to be doing) and some stomach discomfort. There's not a whole lot that you can do about this, other than to drink a lot of water and follow the recommendations below. But trust me: it gets better. And it's absolutely worth it!

Week 1

In weeks 1 and 2, you'll be undergoing what's generally called the "induction phase" in the Atkins Nutritional Approach. This phase will get your body adapted to its new method of metabolism (burning stored fat instead of carbohydrates from food), and because of this it might be the most difficult phase. You're going to be asking your body to make a lot of changes, and that's not always easy. But stick with it! It does get easier, I promise. You're likely to see some pretty good results during this phase, so that should help you stay motivated to stick with it.

To make it easy for you to succeed in this phase, I've taken many of the Atkins rules and summarized them here. I've also included two handy resources at the end of the book: first, a rules guide, in which all of this information is repeated, with lists of all the foods allowed and disallowed in the diet, and the amounts of them that you can eat; and the quick-start guide which I've already mentioned.

1. Eat no more than 20 grams of carbohydrates per day.

This may seem awfully low, but it's what's required to fire up the physiological processes that will turn your body into a fat-burning machine. And when I say "no more than 20 grams," I mean *not a single gram more than 20*. You may think it's alright to have 21 one day, or 22, but don't fall into this trap! I know the story of one woman whose diet was going really well, but she started cheating and didn't quite get her diet back under control until she was back at her original weight.

The key is being absolutely uncompromising when it comes to the 20-gram guideline. You may also hear of diets that use a different number of carbohydrates during the first phase, but these are not Atkins diets, and aren't formulated the same way. So, really, 20 grams, and no more. If you're wondering what 20 grams is, it's about 3 cups of loosely packed salad vegetables, like lettuce, celery, jicama, cucumber, radishes, peppers, or mushrooms. If your intake of salad greens doesn't exceed 2 cups in a day, you can have an additional cup of other vegetables: things like artichoke hearts, onion, kohlrabi, peas, squash, zucchini, kale, pumpkin, and sauerkraut (see the resources at the end of the book for more complete lists).

2. Avoid alcohol, caffeine, and most artificial sweeteners.

I know that this can be tough, but it's quite important to avoid alcohol, caffeine, and all artificial sweeteners other than sucralose (which can be bought under the brand name Splenda). Exactly why this is important gets into the science of fuels and biological processes, but it can all be summed up in the fact that they will keep you out of the fat-burning zone that you're conditioning your body to remain in by cutting out carbohydrates.

3. Start taking nutritional supplements.

Throughout the entirety of this diet, you should be taking a couple nutritional supplements—these will help ensure that you're getting any nutrients that you might be missing out on now that you've cut many foods out of your diet, and will also help you avoid some possible side effects of the first phase, such as leg cramps or gastrointestinal distress. There are two specific supplements that I recommend: a high-quality multivitamin and a fish oil pill for omega 3 fatty acids. You should get these from a health foods store to make sure that you're getting the highest quality supplements you can get; if you just pick up a bottle or two from the corner grocery store, you may not receive the full benefits.

Week 2

The second week of the diet is the same as the first—continue with your carbohydrate restriction and supplementation, and keep avoiding the foods on the restricted list. Hopefully by now things should be getting a little easier. The cravings should be subsiding a bit, any withdrawal symptoms you experienced should be going away, and your weight loss should be fired up.

Unfortunately, this is around the time when many people start to cheat. Even if the pounds are flying off, *don't cheat*. This is the most important part of the diet; during these first two weeks, your body establishes a state of ketosis, and there's no way that you can be "mostly" or "almost" in ketosis—you either are or you aren't. So if you're cheating or not quite abiding by the rules, you're not going to be making the physiological changes that are required for effective and sustained weight loss.

Week two is a great time to start exercising, if it's not something that you do on a regular basis already. If your body is having a hard time adjusting to the diet, you may not want to exercise, but it's actually quite likely to make you feel better. No matter how you're feeling, though, you should start adding exercise to your routine (see section 3.4 for more information on exercise, why it's important, and how to go about starting it).

Week 3

Once you've made it through the first two weeks, you can transition to "ongoing weight loss," the second phase of the Atkins diet. In this phase, you'll still be losing weight, just not quite as quickly as before. Beginning this week, you'll start increasing your carbohydrate intake gradually until you find the level at which you're losing weight slowly, but steadily. Again, the exact rate of weight loss that you're comfortable with is up to you. The increased carbohydrate allowance is what makes ongoing weight loss easier than the induction phase for many people.

It's possible to stay in the induction phase longer than two weeks if you don't need the added carbohydrates, but I generally recommend staying in it for only fourteen days, as more time at 20 grams per day can be difficult and make you consider cheating.

In the ongoing weight loss phase, you will continue eating from the same carbohydrate groups, but you can add a few other sources as well. You should add them slowly, and in a specific order (see step #2 below), but it can be really nice to have some added variety in your diet! Be careful when starting this phase—it can be easy to want to cheat now that you're eating more carbohydrates, but stay within the guidelines or you might find that your weight loss slows significantly or even goes in reverse.

1. Add 5 grams of carbohydrate to your allowance each week.

On the week after your final week of the induction phase, you can have 25 grams of carbohydrate per day. The week after that, you can have 30 grams each day. After that, 35. And so on. In general, people will lose weight in proportion to their carbohydrate restriction, meaning that the more carbohydrates you consume, the more your weight loss will slow.

So, with this information in mind, you should keep increasing the amount of carbohydrate that you consume each day until you reach a point where you're comfortable both with your intake and your weight loss. For some people, this will be 35 grams per day. For others, it might be 50. It varies a lot, and there isn't a specific number that you should be aiming for here. It's totally up to you. If you're really unsure about what you should be aiming for, I'd recommend increasing your carbohydrate intake until you're losing somewhere between one-half and one pound per week.

2. Add carbohydrates in the right order.

Certain carbohydrates are more conducive to weight loss than others, and because your body's gotten used to being on such a low number per day, you should be careful when adding them back into your diet. Fortunately, Dr. Atkins came up with a "carbohydrate pyramid" that will give you some guidance as to which carb sources you should add to your diet in which order. Here's the list:

- More salad and other vegetables on the acceptable foods list
- Fresh cheeses (as well as more aged cheese)
- Seeds and nuts
- Berries
- Wine and other spirits low in carbs
- Legumes
- Fruits other than berries and melons
- Starchy vegetables
- Whole grains

As you can see, the first few items on the list are things you've already been eating, but you'll now be able to have more and a slightly wider variety. After that, you get into foods that are prohibited during the induction phase, which can be a real treat! Again, though, be wary of over-indulging. How fast you add these things to your diet is up to you, but I wouldn't go more than one step on the pyramid each week. In fact, staying at each one for at least two weeks would probably be better, if you're able. Again, it depends largely on your level of comfort with your diet and your current rate of weight loss.

The first three weeks of the diet are likely to be the hardest, but once you make it to this point, you'll be well on your way to becoming a fat-burning machine!

3.3. Managing hormones

As I mentioned in section 2.2, there are two hormones that are of crucial importance when it comes to weight loss: insulin and cortisol. And by managing both of them, you can not only set yourself up for success in your weight loss endeavors, but also help reduce the risk of serious issues and conditions down the road. This section will go over the basics of managing your hormone levels, which is a facet of dieting that is often overlooked.

1. Insulin.

Insulin and abdominal fat are closely related—as insulin rises, more fat is stored around the organs in your abdomen. And as this process continues, your body becomes less and less sensitive to insulin, resulting in more carbohydrate consumption, which causes the release of more insulin. It's a cycle that you need to break out of. I'll outline three different strategies here that will help you fight insulin resistance and help you keep your hormonal responses to food under control.

First, avoid all added sugars. This is absolutely crucial—food products that contain high amounts of added sugar, like candies, processed and pre-packaged foods, and many baked goods, will send your blood sugar skyrocketing, which will result in a huge increase in the amount of insulin in your blood. So when you're choosing the carbohydrates that you'll eat to get to your daily quota, make sure that you're not choosing items like these.

If you need to sweeten something, use a more natural sweetener, like honey or a small amount of stevia. This isn't going to be easy at first—I know how hard it is to kick a sugar habit, and I'm not going to tell you that it's a quick and easy process. But it can be done, and you will glad you did it, especially when you see the pounds and inches coming off.

Second, consume low-GI meals as often as possible. This is actually pretty easy to do when you cut out most carbohydrates, as you'll be left with mostly protein and fat, two nutrients that lower the glycemic index of the foods they're consumed with. Another way to make sure that your blood sugar stays under control is by adding good sources of fiber to your diet. In case you're not sure where to get fiber, here's a list from WebMD of the ten most fiber-rich foods:

- Beans
- Whole grains
- Brown rice
- Popcorn
- Nuts
- Baked potato with skin
- Berries
- Bran cereal
- Oatmeal
- Vegetables

It can be hard to get a lot of fiber when you're cutting out carbohydrates, so it's important to select any available foods from this list for your carbohydrate intake as often as possible. If you're finding it hard to get to your daily recommendation of 25 grams for women (38 grams for men), you might consider taking a fiber supplement, like FiberChoice or Metamucil. Fiber is hugely important, so don't neglect it. If you're not getting enough, try to find a way to increase your intake!

Finally, you can manage your insulin by eating smaller meals more often during the day. When you consume a smaller number of calories, your blood sugar doesn't go up as drastically, and your body doesn't need to release as much insulin. You can use this to your advantage by consuming four or five smaller meals throughout the day instead of three larger ones. This takes a bit of getting used to, but you might find that you like it a lot more than the traditional three-meals-per-day schedule, especially if you find that you often get a mid-afternoon energy slump (I certainly do if I only eat three times in a day).

2. Cortisol.

You may remember that cortisol is released during times of mental or physical stress, and that it increases the amount of fat stored around the abdomen. However, you may not be aware of all the things that qualify as "stress" and contribute to the buildup of cortisol in the body. For example, not getting enough sleep can cause the release of cortisol. So if you're not getting seven to eight hours of sleep every night, you could be contributing to an increase in abdominal fat without even knowing it! By getting adequate amounts of sleep and getting to bed around the same time every night, you'll help keep your body functioning properly.

Another thing that can cause cortisol release is related to the points I brought up just a moment ago: not eating often enough! It seems strange that eating more often can actually help you lose weight, but there's solid scientific evidence that if you eat the right foods at the right times, you can eat more often than you think and still lose weight.

One method that you can use to get your cortisol in line is one that I feel very strongly about: stress management. Many people don't realize that prolonged (chronic) stress can be very detrimental to their health, especially if they're trying to lose weight. But taking care of yourself is hugely important. Everyone has their own preferred method of stress management, but there are a few that I can suggest here that many people find to be helpful.

First, take time to get away. It doesn't need to be much—schedule a day at the spa for yourself, or go down to the corner coffee shop to sit with a few hours with a book and a latte. Schedule a massage or an acupuncture session (acupuncture is actually one of my personal favorites!). It doesn't need to be much—sometimes just going for a walk by yourself for half an hour is enough to clear your mind and help you relax. As long as you're setting time aside for yourself, and not worrying about all of the things that stress you out in everyday life, it'll be well worth the time and effort. Put this on your calendar! It's something that a lot of people find difficult to do, because they feel like they're neglecting important things, but you need to remember that it'll help you meet your weight loss goals and improve your health.

Second, use exercise as a stress reliever. I know this might sound crazy if you think that exercise is always really hard and unpleasant work, but if you stick with it you'll see what I mean. I know several people who feel better about absolutely everything after they've gone on a hard run. But it doesn't need to be training for a marathon—go lift weights for half an hour, or get on the elliptical for a bit, or even do 20 minutes of stretching over your lunch break. Moving your body can really clear your mind!

Finally, learn to say "no." This is definitely the hardest recommendation I have when it comes to stress relief, even if it sounds pretty easy. But our society places a huge value on being busy all the time and feeling productive, and many people embrace this to a fault. For example, if your boss asked you to take on an extra project at work, what would you say? Would you consider your current workload, or would you just say yes, because you want to impress them with how much work you can accomplish? Yes, that extra project might make it a little bit more likely that you'll be the one to get a raise or a promotion, but it may also have consequences for your mental health (and, as we've seen, your physical health as well). This is most evident in people's professional lives, which we often place above our personal and social ones. Learn to say no, spend more time with your family and friends, and take care of yourself. You'll be amazed at how much better you feel. You might even find that you're able to get more work done because you're not feeling stressed or getting sick all the time. Give it a shot—you might be surprised!

3.4. Exercise

No matter which diet you're on, and what your weight loss goals are, exercise is an absolutely indispensable tool that will help you get there. Earlier in the book, I mentioned the link between calories and energy. Well, when your muscles and organs need energy for activity (like when you're exercising), they're going to burn a lot of calories. And because the calorie deficit is the most important thing in any diet, exercising can only be to your advantage. It burns calories; increases your metabolism, even after you're done exercising; builds muscle, further increasing your metabolism; helps manage your hormones; and improves your overall health by strengthening your muscles and bones as well as increasing your cardiovascular fitness. Regular exercise is not a "plus" on a diet, it's a necessity.

The CDC recommends 2 hours and 30 minutes of moderate-intensity aerobic exercise per week. That workouts out to 30 minutes of exercise, five days a week. To help you get there, I've condensed my exercise suggestions (which could fill up a book in their own right) into four simple points.

1. Try new things.

Trying something new is a really fun way to meet new people and get exercise, and many people find it much more motivating than just going to the gym to hit the weights or spend time on the treadmill (there's a reason that runners call it the "dreadmill"). Try tennis, take an aerobics class, or start some weightlifting (if you're feeling quite athletic, try kettlebells or a class like BodyPump). When I moved to a new city recently, I joined a mountain biking group, and I've met people and gotten to explore the surrounding area—it's definitely a great way to get to learn a new place. Try out a bunch of different things and see what you like! You never know what you might discover. I've introduced several people to lap swimming, and they've been surprised at how much they enjoy it. I can even give you a personal example: for a very long time, I thought that I would never enjoy dancing, but my wife got me into swing dancing a few years ago, and it's become one of my favorite activities. (Lindy hop, by the way, is a fantastic and really fun way to exercise!)

2. Make exercise a part of your life.

We are hopelessly tied to our computers and mobile phones, but you can actually turn this to your advantage when it comes to exercise. Plan the exercise that you're going to do for the week, and add it to your calendar (I've used both iCal and Google Calendar for this, and they both work great). If you see that there's a workout coming up and it's on your calendar, you'll be less likely to skip it. This also serves to help you to remember that you need to exercise in the first place! A woman that I know tried to lose weight during graduate school, and she found that she was so busy that she just forgot to exercise on some days. By using this strategy, she was able to make sure that she scheduled time for her workouts. If you have an exercise partner (see the next tip), you can share calendar events so that there's less of a chance that either of you will back out of meeting up to exercise.

3. Get an exercise partner.

One of the most motivating things that you can do is to agree with a family member, friend, or co-worker to exercise together on a regular basis. Maybe you can set up a weekly date with your spouse to go for a bike ride, or go to the gym twice a week with one of your co-workers. Whoever you find, and whatever you decide to do, make sure that you hold each other accountable! It's much more difficult to skip a workout when you have to admit to someone that your shirked your responsibility, and it's even more difficult if you know that they're waiting for you down in the lobby.

4. Track your progress.

Just like with weight loss, keeping track of how far you've come with exercise can be really helpful. If you start jogging, for example, and you start out being able to go for 10 minutes, it can feel like your goal of running a 10k is really far away. But if you keep working at it, before you know it, you'll be going for 20 minutes, and then 25, and then 30, and pretty soon you'll be running for a full hour! If you decide to take a yoga class, you might struggle with some of the poses, but after a while, you'll find that they get significantly easier. Whatever you're doing to get your heart rate up, give yourself some credit for the advances you make. You're getting more fit, you're burning a bunch of calories, and you're improving your overall health. You deserve some credit!

3.5. What to do next

Once you get within about 5 pounds of your goal weight, it's time to switch into the third phase, pre-maintenance. You can think of this as a training phase for the final step, lifetime maintenance. Your goal here is to slow your weight loss down significantly and get used to the type of diet that you'll be on that will help you maintain your goal weight for the rest of your life (which is a pretty exciting thought, isn't it?). In *Dr. Atkins' New Diet Revolution*, Dr. Atkins stresses the importance of this phase, and makes it very clear that this is a crucial step on the way to permanent weight loss, and that it absolutely should not be skipped. When you only have 5 pounds or so to lose, it can be easy to think that you should just stick with an earlier phase and get rid of them in a couple weeks, but there's a very good reason that you should instead slow down drastically. The way you eat to lose weight and the way that you eat to maintain your weight are quite different, and this phase provides some really good practice for maintaining your weight. In fact, many people find it beneficial to enter this phase when they have as many as 15 or 20 pounds left to lose, and to go through those pounds very slowly. I certainly understand wanting to get to your goal quickly, but remember that what you really want to do is get to your goal weight and *stay there*. The pre-maintenance phase is about learning to stay there. Dr. Atkins recommends spending at least one month (two or three, ideally) in this phase.

1. Speed up your carbohydrate increase.

Like the ongoing weight loss phase, you'll be increasing your carbohydrate intake each week. This time, however, you should increase it by 10 grams per week instead of 5 grams. You can keep this going until you're losing less than a pound a week. One pound every two or even every three weeks is a good rate to aim for. I'll stress again that I know that you'll want to keep going at a faster rate than this, but it's absolutely crucial that you don't.

2. Be prepared for some difficulties.

I'm going to be honest with you here: this phase can be tough. As your carb intake increases further, you might start to feel some cravings again, likely for simple sugars and sweets. You can overcome these by using the discipline that you've developed over the past several weeks and months of weight loss. You know how to eat healthily now, and you know what your body feels like when your diet is on track. Keep these feelings in mind, and don't get sidetracked. If you encounter a plateau during this phase, just stick with the plan—slowing your carbohydrate increase and increasing your weekly exercise should be very helpful in getting you over this particular obstacle.

3. Pay close attention.

As in the ongoing weight loss phase, you can be adding new foods very slowly to your diet. You should pay attention to how each food affects you—does it provoke weight gain? Does it cause you digestive difficulty? If there's a food that seems to be messing with your body, take it out of your diet immediately. Some foods might also increase your hunger level or your cravings, and these are foods that you should get rid of as soon as possible. This is a skill that will benefit you greatly in the long run, while you're working to maintain your goal weight. If you start gaining weight again, you can decrease your carbohydrate intake by 5 or 10 grams for a week or two to stop the slide.

I've given you several warnings here, but don't be too worried—this phase is actually a really great one, because you get to experiment with different foods and start laying the foundation for lifelong maintenance of your ideal weight! By now, you'll have lost a significant portion of the weight that you set out to lose at the beginning of the diet, and you're closing in on your goal, and now it's time to make sure that you get there and stay there. As I mentioned, you should spend quite a bit of time in this stage before moving onto the final stage of the diet.

The final stage of the Atkins diet is called "lifetime maintenance." Calling this the "final stage" is a bit misleading, because it makes it sound like it's the end of your diet when, in fact, it's only the beginning of the rest of your life! The entire diet progression up to this stage has taken you from your previous "normal" diet, through the intense carbohydrate restriction of the induction phase, the slightly less strict ongoing weight loss stage, and the pre-maintenance phase, which got you ready for this step. Lifetime maintenance is just like it sounds—maintaining your goal weight for the rest of your life. Because just getting down to your goal isn't enough: you actually have to *stay* there for the diet to be a success. You've gradually worked toward this stage, and now you've made it!

1. Use the knowledge you gained in the pre-maintenance phase.

This point is actually two-fold. The first piece of information that you need to use is the number of carbohydrates that you can consume in a day without gaining weight. Maybe you found you could eat 35 grams, and maybe you found you could eat 55 grams. Whatever that number is, this is the number that you should be aiming for every day. This is the single most important number in the maintenance of your weight over the coming years, and it's one that you should keep in mind when you're planning your diet. By keeping your carbohydrate intake at the maintenance level (what Dr. Atkins calls the "critical carbohydrate level for maintenance"), you'll help keep your weight stable around your ideal weight—of course, you'll have a few ups and downs now and then, but if you stick to your plan, you shouldn't have too much of a problem. The second type of knowledge that you need to keep using is the list of foods and habits that you discovered during the pre-maintenance phase. Keep avoiding the foods that give you cravings or cause you some gastronomic distress, and stick with the foods that seem to work well for you. It's possible that these foods will change, but in general, these are going to be rules that you'll have to continue following.

2. Continue to monitor your progress.

Dr. Atkins recommends weighing yourself once a week during this phase. I prefer to suggest once every two weeks, but you can do whatever works for you. The object of weighing in regularly is to make sure that you keep track of your progress, and so that you're reminded on a regular basis of your motivation for sticking to the maintenance plan. You should aim to always be within 5 pounds of your goal weight. If you get to more than 5 pounds above your goal, you should start up on the induction or ongoing weight loss phase strategies for a week or two to get back down to where you should be. Don't compromise on this—if you find that you're 6 or 7 pounds above your goal weight, don't just say "oh well, I'm close to the 5-pound mark, I'll just get back down in a week." This is the kind of thinking that will cause your weight to creep back up! Be very strict about the 5-pound rule.

3. Adapt the plan to your life.

For the most part, the Atkins Nutritional Approach is a pretty flexible plan, and this is especially true in the lifetime maintenance phase. Obviously, there will be times where it's really hard to stick to the exact numbers that you've set out (I find that this is especially true around the holidays!). However, that doesn't mean you're off the hook: it just means that you have to do a little planning. For example, if you know that you're going to be at a holiday party and that you're likely to consume more carbohydrates than your plan allows for, aim to consume fewer carbs in the days leading up to the party. If this is a plan that you're going to be successfully using for the rest of your life, you'll need to learn how to adapt it to cope with unexpected circumstances.

And there you have it—the progression of the entire Atkins Nutritional Approach! You'll go from the induction phase in day one to lifetime maintenance, which will help you maintain your ideal weight for the rest of your life—it's a lot of work, and it takes a long time, but it's worth it.

4. Resources

In this section, I've included two resources that I think you'll find very useful in your weight-loss endeavors. The first is a quick-start guide that sums up some of the basics of weight loss as well as the first steps of the diet, and provides exercise recommendations. Basically, it's the short-form guide to weight loss with the Atkins diet. The second resource is a list of foods that are allowed or prohibited in each phase of the diet, as well as information on how you should be adjusting your carbohydrate intake throughout the weight-loss process. I hope that you find these helpful—feel free to photocopy them and put them in your kitchen or give them to friends who are curious about using Atkins to get rid of abdominal fat!

4.1. Quick-start guide

1. Set your goal weight.

At what weight did you last feel and look great? This is a good weight to aim for. You can also ask a physician or a personal trainer, who can give you informed advice. Make sure to monitor your progress toward this goal on a regular basis (preferably at least once a week).

2. Begin the induction phase.

Cut your daily carbohydrate intake down to 20 grams, which is about three loosely packed cups of salad vegetables like lettuce, jicama, cabbage, cucumbers and peppers. These are the only carbohydrates you should be eating. Consume high-quality sources of protein and fat to make sure you're getting enough calories each day. Stay in this phase for a minimum of two weeks.

3. Decide when you're ready to move to step 2.

The ongoing weight loss phase starts when you feel you're ready to move. Whether you're bored with the induction phase or having a lot of difficulty with it, moving to the next phase can be very helpful.

4. Keep weight loss moving.

During the second phase, ongoing weight loss, add 5 grams to your daily intake each week. Most of this should come from salad vegetables, but you can start adding a few other vegetables back into your diet, and after several weeks, some other sources of carbohydrates.

5. Prepare for the rest of your life.

The pre-maintenance phase should start when you're approaching your goal weight, usually when you're within 5 or 10 pounds. Your carbohydrate intake can speed up to 10 grams per day per week, until you're losing weight very slowly. Continue this until you're at your goal weight.

6. Enter the maintenance phase.

Once you've reached your goal weight and discovered the number of carbohydrates you can consume without gaining weight, you're ready to plan for the future. Keep consuming this amount of carbohydrates, and you should stay at your goal weight for a long time!

7. Go back to earlier phases if needed.

If you start gaining weight again, go back to the induction or ongoing weight loss phase for a couple weeks to get back to where you should be (you should do this once you've hit five pounds above your goal weight).

8. Exercise!

Exercise is hugely important, so don't neglect it. Aim for at least 30 minutes, five days a week.

4.2. Food lists

1. Allowable vegetables during the induction phase (20 grams per day).

- alfalfa sprouts
- arugula
- bok choy
- celery
- chicory
- chives
- cucumber
- daikon
- mushrooms
- endive
- parsley
- escarole
- peppers
- fennel
- radicchio
- jicama
- radishes
- lettuce
- romaine
- mache
- sorrel

2. Other acceptable vegetables for the induction phase (should make up no more than a third of your carb intake).

- artichoke hearts
- asparagus
- bamboo shoots
- bean sprouts

- beet greens
- broccoli
- broccoli rabe
- brussels sprouts
- cabbage
- cauliflower
- celery root (celeriac)
- chard
- collard greens
- dandelion greens
- eggplant
- hearts of palm
- kale
- kohlrabi
- leeks
- okra
- onion
- pumpkin
- rhubarb
- sauerkraut
- scallions
- snow peas
- spaghetti squash
- spinach
- string or wax beans
- summer squash
- tomato
- turnips
- water chestnuts
- zucchini

3. The carbohydrate ladder (when you start adding more carbohydrates to your diet, start at #1 and move slowly toward #9).

- More salad and other vegetables on the acceptable foods list
- Fresh cheeses (as well as more aged cheese)

- Seeds and nuts
- Berries
- Wine and other spirits low in carbs
- Legumes
- Fruits other than berries and melons
- Starchy vegetables
- Whole grains

73 Savory Fat Burning Recipes

BREAKFAST

1. Luscious Berry Smoothie

Servings: 4
Ready in: 8 minutes

Nutrition Facts

Serving Size 127 g

Amount Per Serving	
Calories 86	Calories from Fat 38
	% Daily Value*
Total Fat 4.3g	**7%**
Trans Fat 0.0g	
Cholesterol 0mg	**0%**
Sodium 20mg	**1%**
Total Carbohydrates 5.6g	**2%**
Dietary Fiber 5.6g	**22%**
Sugars 3.1g	
Protein 4.4g	
Vitamin A 1% •	Vitamin C 36%
Calcium 8% •	Iron 5%

Nutrition Grade B

* Based on a 2000 calorie diet

Ingredients

- 3/4 cup sliced fresh strawberries
- 1/2 cup fresh sliced raspberries
- 5 whole almonds
- 1 cup ice cubes
- 1/2 cup pure organic soy milk
- 1/2 teaspoon ground cinnamon
- 1 teaspoon pure vanilla extract

- 1/4 cup flax seeds

Directions

Combine all ingredients in a blender and puree until smooth.

2. No Crust Spinach N' Mushroom Quiche

Servings: 5
Preparation time: 10 minutes
Cook time: 40 minutes
Ready in: 50 minutes

Nutrition Facts

Serving Size 196 g

Amount Per Serving

Calories 364   Calories from Fat 251

	% Daily Value*
Total Fat 27.9g	**43%**
Saturated Fat 14.7g	**74%**
Cholesterol 224mg	**75%**
Sodium 556mg	**23%**
Total Carbohydrates 5.3g	**2%**
Dietary Fiber 1.7g	**7%**
Sugars 2.0g	
Protein 24.1g	

Vitamin A 101%	*	Vitamin C 28%
Calcium 58%	*	Iron 16%

Nutrition Grade B
* Based on a 2000 calorie diet

Ingredients
- 1 tablespoon olive oil, plus extra amount for greasing
- 1 clove garlic, minced
- 1 medium onion, chopped
- 1/2 cup sliced mushrooms
- 1 (8 ounce) package frozen chopped spinach, thawed and drained
- 5 (omega-3) eggs, beaten
- 3 cups shredded Monterey Jack cheese
- 2 teaspoons chopped fresh basil leaves
- 2 green onions, minced
- 1/4 teaspoon sea salt

- 1/8 teaspoon ground black pepper

Directions

1. **Preheat** oven to 350 degrees F (175 degrees C). Grease a 9 inch pie pan with olive oil.
2. **Place** a large skillet over medium-high heat; pour olive oil into the skillet. Once the oil is hot, add the garlic, onion, and mushrooms; stir and cook, until onion is soft.
3. **Stir** in spinach and cook until wilted.
4. **Whisk** together the eggs, cheese, basil leaves, green onions, salt, and pepper in a large bowl. Stir in the cooked spinach mixture and then place mixture into the prepared pie pan.
5. **Bake** for about 30 minutes, or until set. Cool and serve.

3. Bacon and Cheese Deviled Eggs

Servings: 6
Preparation time: 15 minutes
Cook time: 15 minutes
Ready in: 30 minutes

Nutrition Facts

Serving Size 83 g

Amount Per Serving

Calories 218	Calories from Fat 152

	% Daily Value*
Total Fat 16.9g	**26%**
Saturated Fat 4.3g	**22%**
Trans Fat 0.0g	
Cholesterol 184mg	**61%**
Sodium 657mg	**27%**
Total Carbohydrates 5.8g	**2%**
Sugars 1.7g	
Protein 11.1g	

Vitamin A 9%	•	Vitamin C 4%
Calcium 4%	•	Iron 7%

Nutrition Grade C-
* Based on a 2000 calorie diet

Ingredients

- 6 (omega-3) eggs
- 1/2 cup light mayonnaise
- 4 slices bacon
- 2 tablespoons shredded Cheddar cheese
- 1 tablespoon mustard
- 1/2 cup chopped chives
- 1/2 teaspoon sea salt
- 1/4 teaspoon ground black pepper

Directions

1. **Place** eggs in a saucepan covered with water. Bring water to a boil then remove pan from heat. Let the eggs sit in the hot water for 10 minutes.

2. **Remove** eggs from pan and cool in cold water. Peel and cut in half lengthwise.

3. **Place** a large skillet over medium-high heat. Add bacon and cook until evenly browned. Crumble and set aside.

4. **Remove** egg yolks and place in a medium bowl. Mash the egg yolks with the mayonnaise, cooked bacon and cheese.

5. **Add** the mustard, chives, salt, and pepper; blend well. Fill egg white halves with the yolk mixture. Chill and serve.

4. Breakfast Pork Patties

Servings: 3
Preparation time: 10 minutes
Cook time: 18 minutes
Ready in: 28 minutes

Nutrition Facts

Serving Size 239 g

Amount Per Serving

Calories 483   Calories from Fat 309

% Daily Value*

Total Fat 34.3g	**53%**
Cholesterol 0mg	**0%**
Sodium 1250mg	**52%**
Total Carbohydrates 5.4g	**2%**
Dietary Fiber 0.9g	**4%**
Sugars 3.9g	
Protein 39.0g	

Vitamin A 4%	Vitamin C 2%
Calcium 3%	Iron 4%

Nutrition Grade D+

* Based on a 2000 calorie diet

Ingredients
- 1/4 cup chopped fresh basil leaves
- 2 teaspoons dried sage
- 1/2 teaspoon dried rosemary
- 1/4 teaspoon dried marjoram
- 1/8 teaspoon ground cayenne pepper
- 1 1/2 teaspoons fennel seeds
- 2 teaspoons sea salt
- 1 teaspoon ground black pepper
- 2 teaspoons raw honey
- 1 1/2 pounds lean ground pork
- Olive oil for greasing

Directions

1. **Place** ground pork in a large bowl.
2. **Mix** together the basil, sage, rosemary, marjoram, cayenne pepper, fennel seeds, salt, black pepper, and honey in a small bowl.
3. **Add** herb mixture to the pork and mix well. Wet your hands with water and shape mixture into patties.
4. **Grease** a large skillet with olive oil and place over medium high heat.
5. **Sauté** the patties in oil for 5 minutes per side, or until evenly browned.

5. Turkey Breakfast Sausage

Servings: 3
Preparation time: 15 minutes
Cook time: 10 minutes
Ready in: 25 minutes

Nutrition Facts

Serving Size 167 g

Amount Per Serving

Calories 262   Calories from Fat 140

	% Daily Value*
Total Fat 15.6g	**24%**
Saturated Fat 4.1g	**20%**
Trans Fat 0.0g	
Cholesterol 107mg	**36%**
Sodium 1363mg	**57%**
Total Carbohydrates 5.7g	**2%**
Protein 29.8g	

Vitamin A 3%	•	Vitamin C 2%
Calcium 4%	•	Iron 16%

Nutrition Grade D

* Based on a 2000 calorie diet

Ingredients

- 1 teaspoons ground sage
- 1 tablespoon Stevia
- 2 teaspoons sea salt
- 1 teaspoon ground black pepper
- 2 cloves garlic, chopped

- 1/4 teaspoon dried thyme
- 1/2 teaspoon crushed red pepper flakes
- 1/8 teaspoon nutmeg
- 1 1/2 teaspoon dried tarragon
- 1 pound lean ground turkey
- olive oil for greasing

Directions

1. **Mix** all ingredients, except the olive oil, in a large bowl.
2. **Shape** mixture into patties.
3. **Grease** a large skillet with the olive oil and place over medium high heat.
4. **Fry** the patties in the skillet until they are no longer pink inside and internal temperature reaches 160 degrees F, about 5 minutes each side.

6. Cauliflower Hash Browns with Bacon

Servings: 4
Preparation time: 10 minutes
Cook time: 10 minutes
Ready in: 20 minutes

Nutrition Facts

Serving Size 150 g

Amount Per Serving

Calories 250	Calories from Fat 164

	% Daily Value*
Total Fat 18.2g	**28%**
Saturated Fat 7.6g	**38%**
Trans Fat 0.0g	
Cholesterol 87mg	**29%**
Sodium 994mg	**41%**
Total Carbohydrates 6.5g	**2%**
Dietary Fiber 2.4g	**10%**
Sugars 2.7g	
Protein 15.5g	

Vitamin A 5%	•	Vitamin C 68%
Calcium 8%	•	Iron 6%

Nutrition Grade C-
* Based on a 2000 calorie diet

Ingredients
- 1/2 medium head fresh cauliflower, grated
- 1 egg, beaten
- 4 slices bacon, chopped
- 1/2 cup chopped onion
- 1/4 cup cheddar cheese
- 1/2 teaspoon sea salt
- 1/4 teaspoon ground black pepper
- 1 tablespoon melted butter

Directions
1. **Combine** the cauliflower, egg, bacon, onion, cheese, salt and pepper. Shape mixture into several patties.
2. **Heat** butter in a pan over medium high heat.

3. **Add** the patties and cook for about 5 minutes or until browned on both sides.

7. Coconut Almond Pancakes

Servings: 6
Preparation time: 5 minutes
Cook time: 10 minutes
Ready in: 15 minutes

Nutrition Facts

Serving Size 44 g

Amount Per Serving

Calories 146   Calories from Fat 105

% **Daily Value***

Total Fat 11.7g	**18%**
Saturated Fat 3.1g	**16%**
Trans Fat 0.0g	
Cholesterol 55mg	**18%**
Sodium 100mg	**4%**
Total Carbohydrates 7.1g	**2%**
Dietary Fiber 2.3g	**9%**
Sugars 3.9g	
Protein 5.5g	

Vitamin A 1%	•	Vitamin C 1%
Calcium 5%	•	Iron 6%

Nutrition Grade B+

* Based on a 2000 calorie diet

Ingredients
- 2 (omega-3) eggs
- 1/4 cup coconut milk
- 1 tablespoon raw honey
- 1 cup almond meal
- 1/2 teaspoon ground cinnamon
- 1/4 teaspoon sea salt
- coconut oil for greasing

Directions
1. **Beat** together the eggs, coconut milk, and honey in a medium bowl until frothy.
2. **Mix** the almond meal, cinnamon, and salt in a large bowl. Pour the egg mixture into the almond meal mixture.

3. **Grease** a pan with coconut oil then place over medium-low heat. Pour batter (about 3 tablespoons per pancake) onto pan.
4. **Cook** both sides for 2-3 minutes. Serve warm.

8. Spicy Veggie Omelet

Servings: 4
Preparation time: 12 minutes
Cook time: 15 minutes
Ready in: 27 minutes

Nutrition Facts

Serving Size 159 g

Amount Per Serving

Calories 185	Calories from Fat 128

% Daily Value*

Total Fat 14.2g	**22%**
Saturated Fat 5.3g	**27%**
Trans Fat 0.0g	
Cholesterol 92mg	**31%**
Sodium 401mg	**17%**
Total Carbohydrates 7.5g	**3%**
Dietary Fiber 2.0g	**8%**
Sugars 3.9g	
Protein 8.9g	

Vitamin A 23%	•	Vitamin C 81%
Calcium 14%	•	Iron 10%

Nutrition Grade B
* Based on a 2000 calorie diet

Ingredients
- 2 tablespoons olive oil
- 1 clove garlic, minced
- 1 medium onion, chopped
- 2 teaspoons finely chopped jalapeno pepper
- 1 red bell pepper, chopped
- 1 cup sliced mushrooms
- 2 (omega-3) eggs
- 2 tablespoons coconut milk
- 1/2 teaspoon sea salt
- 1/4 teaspoon freshly ground black pepper
- 2 ounces shredded Parmesan cheese
- 1 medium red tomato, diced

Directions

1. **Heat** 1 tablespoon olive oil in a medium skillet over medium heat. Add the garlic and sauté until golden browned.

2. **Stir** in the onion, jalapeno pepper, bell pepper, and mushrooms; cook for 5 minutes, or until just tender. Remove vegetables from pan and set aside.

3. **Beat** together the eggs, milk, salt, and pepper in a medium bowl.

4. **Heat** the remaining 1 tablespoon of olive oil in the same skillet over medium heat. Pour in the egg mixture and cook for 4 minutes, or until set.

5. **Spoon** the cooked vegetables into the center of the omelet. Add the diced tomato then sprinkle with cheese.

6. **Gently** fold one edge of the omelet over the vegetables using a spatula. Cook omelet for another 2 minutes or until the cheese melts to your desired consistency.

7. **Place** omelet onto a plate, slice and serve.

9. Dijonnaise Tuna Breakfast Salad

Servings: 5
Ready in: 15 minutes

Nutrition Facts

Serving Size 86 g

Amount Per Serving

Calories 206	Calories from Fat 132

	% Daily Value*
Total Fat 14.7g	**23%**
Saturated Fat 1.9g	**9%**
Cholesterol 12mg	**4%**
Sodium 571mg	**24%**
Total Carbohydrates 7.5g	**3%**
Dietary Fiber 0.7g	**3%**
Sugars 2.2g	
Protein 12.0g	

Vitamin A 4%	•	Vitamin C 1%
Calcium 2%	•	Iron 5%

Nutrition Grade B
* Based on a 2000 calorie diet

Ingredients
- 1/2 cup light mayonnaise
- 1/4 teaspoon curry powder
- 1 tablespoon prepared Dijon mustard
- 1/2 teaspoon sea salt
- 1/4 teaspoon ground black pepper
- 1 (6 ounce) oil-packed tuna
- 1/2 cup celery, diced
- 1/4 cup walnuts, chopped
- 1 shallot, finely chopped
- 1 teaspoon sweet pickle relish
- 4 leaves lettuce

Directions
1. **Whisk** together the mayonnaise, curry powder, mustard, salt, and pepper in a bowl.
2. **Add** the remaining ingredients and toss to coat.
3. **Cover** and chill for 5 minutes.
4. **Serve** with lettuce leaves.

10. Whole Wheat Blueberry Pancakes

Servings: 6
Preparation time: 10 minutes
Cook time: 8 minutes
Ready in: 18 minutes

Nutrition Facts

Serving Size 83 g

Amount Per Serving

Calories 74	Calories from Fat 32

% Daily Value*

Total Fat 3.6g	**5%**
Trans Fat 0.0g	
Cholesterol 28mg	**9%**
Sodium 187mg	**8%**
Total Carbohydrates 7.9g	**3%**
Dietary Fiber 1.2g	**5%**
Sugars 5.5g	
Protein 3.7g	

Vitamin A 3%	•	Vitamin C 2%
Calcium 12%	•	Iron 3%

Nutrition Grade B
* Based on a 2000 calorie diet

Ingredients
- 1 cup almond flour
- 1 1/2 teaspoons baking powder
- 1/2 teaspoon sea salt
- 1 tablespoon flax meal
- 1/2 teaspoon ground cinnamon
- 1 (omega-3) egg
- 1 cup skim milk
- 1 teaspoon pure vanilla extract
- 2 teaspoons raw honey
- 3/4 cup blueberries
- Coconut oil for greasing

Directions
1. **Combine** the flour, baking powder, salt, flax meal, and cinnamon in a medium mixing bowl. In a separate large bowl, beat together the egg, milk, vanilla, and honey.

2. **Add** the flour mixture and stir until just moistened.
3. **Fold** in the blueberries, and stir to incorporate.
4. **Grease** a large, heavy skillet with coconut oil then place over medium heat. Ladle about 1/4 cup of batter onto the pan for each pancake.
5. **Cook** for about 1 1/2 minutes, or until bubbly. Flip over, and continue cooking until golden brown.

11. Breakfast Almond Porridge

Servings: 5
Preparation time: 8 minutes
Cook time: 12 minutes
Ready in: 20 minutes

Nutrition Facts

Serving Size 132 g

Amount Per Serving

Calories 176   Calories from Fat 141

	% Daily Value*
Total Fat 15.6g	**24%**
Saturated Fat 8.1g	**41%**
Trans Fat 0.0g	
Cholesterol 0mg	**0%**
Sodium 8mg	**0%**
Total Carbohydrates 8.0g	**3%**
Dietary Fiber 2.9g	**11%**
Sugars 4.1g	
Protein 3.9g	

Vitamin A 0%	•	Vitamin C 10%
Calcium 5%	•	Iron 7%

Nutrition Grade B
* Based on a 2000 calorie diet

Ingredients
- 3/4 cup light coconut milk
- 3/4 cup almond meal
- 1 1/2 cup water
- 1 teaspoon ground cinnamon
- 1 teaspoon pure maple syrup
- 1 teaspoon raw honey
- 1/4 cup diced strawberries

Directions

1. **Combine** coconut milk, almond meal, and water in a saucepan over medium heat; stirring continuously until smooth.

2. **Stir** in the cinnamon, maple syrup, and honey. Bring to a slow simmer about 3 minutes, or until thick and bubbly.

3. **Ladle** porridge into bowls and top with diced strawberries. Serve warm.

12. Zucchini and Carrot Frittata

Servings: 4
Preparation time: 10 minutes
Cook time: 25 minutes
Ready in: 35 minutes

Nutrition Facts

Serving Size 243 g

Amount Per Serving

Calories 239	Calories from Fat 150

	% Daily Value*
Total Fat 16.7g	**26%**
Saturated Fat 4.3g	**21%**
Trans Fat 0.0g	
Cholesterol 419mg	**140%**
Sodium 370mg	**15%**
Total Carbohydrates 8.2g	**3%**
Dietary Fiber 2.2g	**9%**
Sugars 4.4g	
Protein 15.6g	

Vitamin A 69%	•	Vitamin C 61%
Calcium 9%	•	Iron 21%

Nutrition Grade B+
* Based on a 2000 calorie diet

Ingredients

- 1 1/2 tablespoon olive oil
- 2 cloves garlic, chopped
- 1 zucchini, diced
- 1/2 cup carrots, chopped
- 1/2 red bell pepper, diced
- 1 shallot, chopped
- 1 tablespoon chopped fresh basil

- 5 large omega-3 eggs
- 1/2 teaspoon sea salt
- 1/4 teaspoon freshly ground black pepper
- 1 medium tomato, seeded and chopped

Directions

1. **Heat** olive oil in a medium oven-proof skillet over medium heat. Add garlic and sauté until lightly browned.
2. **Add** zucchini, carrots, red bell pepper, shallot, and basil. Cover and cook for about 6 minutes, or until tender.
3. **Beat** together the eggs, salt, and pepper in a medium bowl until frothy.
4. **Gently** pour egg mixture over vegetable mixture. Add tomatoes and turn heat to medium-low. Cover and cook for 15 minutes.
5. **Preheat** broiler to low. Cook frittata under the broiler for 3 minutes, or until set.
6. **Transfer** to a plate, slice, and serve.

13. Nut and Seeds Cereal

Servings: 5
Preparation time: 10 minutes
Cook time: 5 minutes
Ready in: 15 minutes

Nutrition Facts

Serving Size 144 g

Amount Per Serving

Calories 126	Calories from Fat 89
	% Daily Value*
Total Fat 9.9g	**15%**
Trans Fat 0.0g	
Cholesterol 0mg	**0%**
Sodium 4mg	**0%**
Total Carbohydrates 8.1g	**3%**
Dietary Fiber 4.6g	**18%**
Sugars 2.8g	
Protein 4.9g	

Vitamin A 0%	•	Vitamin C 0%
Calcium 5%	•	Iron 6%

Nutrition Grade C+

* Based on a 2000 calorie diet

Ingredients
- 2 1/2 cups water
- 1/2 cup flax meal
- 1/2 cup raw almonds, coarsely ground
- 1/4 cup raw unsalted sunflower seeds, coarsely ground
- 2 teaspoons raw honey
- 1/2 teaspoon pure vanilla extract

Directions
1. **Place** all the ingredients in a saucepan over medium-high heat.
2. **Bring** to a boil, stirring frequently. Simmer for at least 2 minutes to thicken. Cool slightly
3. **Ladle** into bowls and serve warm.

14. Walnut Banana Waffles

Servings: 6
Preparation time: 10 minutes
Cook time: 20 minutes
Ready in: 30 minutes

Nutrition Facts

Serving Size 67 g

Amount Per Serving

Calories 91	Calories from Fat 52

% Daily Value*

Total Fat 5.8g	**9%**
Saturated Fat 0.6g	**3%**
Trans Fat 0.0g	
Cholesterol 27mg	**9%**
Sodium 179mg	**7%**
Total Carbohydrates 8.2g	**3%**
Dietary Fiber 1.4g	**6%**
Sugars 3.9g	
Protein 3.5g	

Vitamin A 2%	•	Vitamin C 3%
Calcium 10%	•	Iron 4%

Nutrition Grade B+
* Based on a 2000 calorie diet

Ingredients

- 1 1/4 cups almond flour
- 2 teaspoons baking powder
- 1/2 teaspoon sea salt
- 1/2 teaspoon ground cinnamon
- 1 pinch ground nutmeg
- 1 (omega-3) egg
- 1/2 cup vanilla soy milk
- 1 teaspoon pure maple syrup
- 1/3 cup chopped walnuts
- 2 medium ripe bananas, sliced
- Coconut oil spray for greasing

Directions

1. **Preheat** waffle iron. Sift together flour, baking powder, salt, cinnamon, and nutmeg in a large mixing bowl. Add egg, milk, and maple syrup until mixture is smooth.

2. **Grease** a preheated waffle iron with coconut oil spray. Pour 2 tablespoons of batter onto the hot waffle iron.

3. **Sprinkle** with the chopped walnuts and then place 2 slices of banana on top of the batter.

4. **Spoon** another 2 tablespoons of batter on top of the banana.

5. **Cook** waffles until golden brown.

15. Bacon and Green Beans

Servings: 6
Preparation time: 10 minutes
Cook time: 20 minutes
Ready in: 30 minutes

Nutrition Facts

Serving Size 171 g

Amount Per Serving

Calories 165   Calories from Fat 84

	% Daily Value*
Total Fat 9.4g	**14%**
Saturated Fat 0.6g	**3%**
Cholesterol 0mg	**0%**
Sodium 157mg	**7%**
Total Carbohydrates 8.6g	**3%**
Dietary Fiber 4.7g	**19%**
Sugars 3.4g	
Protein 11.1g	

Vitamin A 14%	•	Vitamin C 41%
Calcium 6%	•	Iron 4%

Nutrition Grade B+

* Based on a 2000 calorie diet

Ingredients

- 10 slices nitrite/nitrate free lean bacon, diced
- 2 cloves garlic, crushed
- 1 small red bell pepper, finely chopped
- 2 (10 ounce) packages frozen whole green beans
- 1/2 teaspoon dried cayenne pepper
- 1/2 teaspoon sea salt

- 1/4 teaspoon ground black pepper
- 1/4 cup onion, finely chopped
- 1/2 cup chopped toasted pecans
- 2 teaspoons lemon juice

Directions

1. **Cook** bacon in a large skillet set over medium-high heat until crisp. Remove bacon from pan and drain on paper towels.
2. **Discard** excess grease from the skillet, leaving about 2 tablespoons in the pan.
3. **Sauté** garlic and red bell pepper in the bacon grease over medium-high heat, until garlic is lightly browned.
4. **Stir** in green beans, cayenne pepper, season with salt, pepper; cook for about 10 minutes, or until beans are tender.
5. **Add** the chopped onion halfway through cooking. Stir in the pecans and cooked bacon to the pan.
6. **Drizzle** with lemon juice and toss.

16. Berry Vanilla Crepes

Servings: 7
Preparation time: 15 minutes
Cook time: 15 minutes
Ready in: 30 minutes

Nutrition Facts

Serving Size 119 g

Amount Per Serving

Calories 152	Calories from Fat 104

% Daily Value*

Total Fat 11.5g	**18%**
Saturated Fat 5.9g	**30%**
Trans Fat 0.0g	
Cholesterol 107mg	**36%**
Sodium 190mg	**8%**
Total Carbohydrates 9.7g	**3%**
Dietary Fiber 1.3g	**5%**
Sugars 7.2g	
Protein 2.6g	

Vitamin A 8%	•	Vitamin C 26%
Calcium 11%	•	Iron 3%

Nutrition Grade D+

* Based on a 2000 calorie diet

Ingredients

- 3 (omega-3) egg yolks
- 1 1/4 cups pure coconut milk
- 1 tablespoon pure vanilla extract
- 1 tablespoon raw honey
- 1 cup almond flour
- 1/4 cup melted butter
- 1/2 teaspoon sea salt
- 1/4 teaspoon ground cinnamon
- 1/4 teaspoon nutmeg
- 1 cup fresh strawberries, sliced
- 1 cup fresh blueberries
- Coconut oil for greasing

Directions

1. **Whisk** together the egg yolks, coconut milk, vanilla, and honey in a large bowl.

2. **Add** the almond flour, butter, salt, cinnamon, and nutmeg; whisk thoroughly.

3. **Grease** a crepe pan with coconut oil then place pan over medium heat.

4. **Spread** batter (about 1/4 cup for each crepe) into the pan. Brown crepes on both sides.

5. **Fill** crepes with berries to serve.

17. Bacon and Eggs Benedict

Servings: 6
Preparation time: 15 minutes
Cook time: 30 minutes
Ready in: 45 minutes

Nutrition Facts

Serving Size 98 g

Amount Per Serving

Calories 220   Calories from Fat 128

	% Daily Value*
Total Fat 14.3g	**22%**
Saturated Fat 4.7g	**24%**
Trans Fat 0.0g	
Cholesterol 256mg	**85%**
Sodium 641mg	**27%**
Total Carbohydrates 10.7g	**4%**
Sugars 2.1g	
Protein 15.2g	

Vitamin A 7%	•	Vitamin C 1%
Calcium 8%	•	Iron 8%

Nutrition Grade B-
* Based on a 2000 calorie diet

Ingredients

- 2 (omega-3) egg yolks
- 1/2 cup plain low-fat yogurt
- 1 teaspoon lemon juice
- 1/2 teaspoon prepared Dijon mustard
- 1/4 teaspoon raw honey

- 1/4 teaspoon sea salt
- 1 pinch ground black pepper
- 1/4 teaspoon ground cayenne pepper
- 6 eggs
- 6 slices Pumpernickel bread
- 6 (1-ounce) slices bacon, cut into thin slices
- 1 tablespoon chopped fresh cilantro, for garnish

Directions

1. **Whisk** together the egg yolks, yogurt, lemon juice, mustard, honey, salt, black pepper, and cayenne pepper in the top of a double boiler.
2. **Cook** over simmering water for 6 to 8 minutes, stirring constantly until thick.
3. **Fill** a large stock pot with 2 quarts of salted water. Bring water to a slow boil over medium-high heat.
4. **Gently** break 1 of the eggs into the boiling water; repeat with the remaining eggs. Reduce the heat to medium.
5. **Cook** until the egg white is set, about 3 minutes; remove eggs with a slotted spoon and drain.
6. **Toast** bread slices and place on warm plates. Top each toast with bacon and poached egg. Drizzle with the prepared sauce and sprinkle with cilantro.

18. Flax Pumpkin Bread

Servings: 6
Preparation time: 10 minutes
Cook time: 35 minutes
Ready in: 45 minutes

Nutrition Facts

Serving Size 82 g

Amount Per Serving

Calories 177	Calories from Fat 111

	% Daily Value*
Total Fat 12.4g	**19%**
Saturated Fat 2.9g	**14%**
Trans Fat 0.0g	
Cholesterol 0mg	**0%**
Sodium 191mg	**8%**
Total Carbohydrates 11.4g	**4%**
Dietary Fiber 4.0g	**16%**
Sugars 6.1g	
Protein 5.2g	

Vitamin A 20%	•	Vitamin C 2%
Calcium 2%	•	Iron 2%

Nutrition Grade C

* Based on a 2000 calorie diet

Ingredients

- 3 tablespoons ground flaxseeds
- 1/2 cup water
- 1 cup blanched almond flour
- 1/2 teaspoon baking soda
- 1/2 tablespoon ground cinnamon
- 1 teaspoon ground nutmeg
- 1/4 teaspoon sea salt
- 1/2 cup roasted pumpkin, mashed
- 2 tablespoons raw honey
- coconut oil for greasing

Directions

1. **Preheat** oven to 350 degrees F. Grease a mini loaf pan with coconut oil.

2. **Combine** the ground flaxseeds and water until thick. Set aside. Mix the almond flour, baking soda, cinnamon, nutmeg, and salt in a separate bowl.

3. **Add** flaxseed mixture, pumpkin, and honey; blend well. Pour batter into the prepared loaf pan.

4. **Bake** for 35-45 minutes, or until a toothpick inserted into the center of the bread comes out clean.

19. Easy Fresh Insalata Caprese

Servings: 5
Ready in: 15 minutes

Nutrition Facts

Serving Size 264 g

Amount Per Serving

Calories 380   Calories from Fat 242

                                    % Daily Value*

Total Fat 26.9g	**41%**
Saturated Fat 12.7g	**64%**
Trans Fat 0.0g	
Cholesterol 49mg	**16%**
Sodium 675mg	**28%**
Total Carbohydrates 10.7g	**4%**
Dietary Fiber 2.2g	**9%**
Sugars 4.5g	
Protein 25.3g	

Vitamin A 12%	•	Vitamin C 53%
Calcium 68%	•	Iron 17%

Nutrition Grade B

* Based on a 2000 calorie diet

Ingredients
- 4 large ripe tomatoes, sliced 1/4 inch thick
- 1/3 cup fresh basil leaves
- 1 pound fresh mozzarella cheese, sliced 1/4 inch thick
- 1/2 cup sliced Portobello mushrooms
- 3 cloves garlic, chopped
- 2 teaspoons dried oregano
- 1/2 teaspoon sea salt
- 1/4 ground black pepper
- 3 tablespoons extra virgin olive oil

- 2 tablespoons white balsamic vinegar

Directions
1. **Arrange** the tomato slices, mozzarella cheese slices, mushrooms, and basil leaves on a platter; alternating and overlapping them.
2. **Sprinkle** with chopped garlic and dried oregano then season with salt and pepper.
3. **Drizzle** with olive oil and balsamic vinegar.

20. Asparagus Chicken Stir-Fry

Servings: 4
Preparation time: 10 minutes
Cook time: 15 minutes
Ready in: 25 minutes

Nutrition Facts

Serving Size 290 g

Amount Per Serving

Calories 260   Calories from Fat 108

	% Daily Value*
Total Fat 11.9g	**18%**
Saturated Fat 2.0g	**10%**
Cholesterol 49mg	**16%**
Sodium 1484mg	**62%**
Total Carbohydrates 10.5g	**3%**
Dietary Fiber 4.6g	**18%**
Sugars 6.1g	
Protein 28.5g	

Vitamin A 50%   •   Vitamin C 142%
Calcium 4%   •   Iron 15%

Nutrition Grade B+
* Based on a 2000 calorie diet

Ingredients
- 2 tablespoons olive oil
- 1 pound lean chicken breast, diced
- 2 cloves garlic, minced
- 1/2 lb. asparagus, cut into 1-2" pieces
- 4 medium scallions, thinly sliced
- 2 red bell peppers, sliced
- 1 thumb-size ginger, peeled and julienned

- 1 tablespoon soy sauce
- 1/2 teaspoon sea salt
- 1/2 avocado, sliced

Directions

1. **Heat** 1 tablespoon of olive oil in a large skillet over medium-high heat. Add chicken and fry until thoroughly cooked. Remove to a plate and set aside.
2. **Heat** the remaining 1 tablespoon olive oil in the same skillet. Add garlic, asparagus, scallions, red bell pepper, and ginger; sauté and simmer vegetables for 5 minutes, or until slightly tender.
3. **Stir** in chicken and soy sauce; simmer until heated through then season with salt.
4. **Top** with avocado slices to serve.

21. Low-Carb Granola

Servings: 6
Preparation time: 10 minutes
Cook time: 20 minutes
Ready in: 30 minutes

Nutrition Facts

Serving Size 92 g

Amount Per Serving

Calories 417　　　　Calories from Fat 351

	% Daily Value*
Total Fat 39.0g	**60%**
Saturated Fat 19.2g	**96%**
Trans Fat 0.0g	
Cholesterol 0mg	**0%**
Sodium 163mg	**7%**
Total Carbohydrates 11.1g	**4%**
Dietary Fiber 7.7g	**31%**
Sugars 6.9g	
Protein 8.1g	

Vitamin A 0%	•	Vitamin C 1%
Calcium 6%	•	Iron 14%

Nutrition Grade C+

* Based on a 2000 calorie diet

Ingredients

- 1/2 cup coconut oil
- 3 tablespoons pure maple syrup
- 1 teaspoon ground cinnamon
- 1/2 cup raw walnuts
- 1/2 cup raw pecans
- 1/2 cup shredded coconut, unsweetened
- 1/2 cup sunflower seeds
- 1/2 cup flax seed meal
- 1/2 teaspoon sea salt
- 1/2 cup water

Directions

1. **Preheat** oven to 300 degrees F. Line a baking sheet with parchment paper.
2. **Stir** together the coconut oil, maple syrup, and cinnamon in a medium bowl. Microwave for a few minutes just until warm then let cool slightly.
3. **Combine** the remaining ingredients with the coconut oil mixture; stir to coat. Spread mixture evenly onto the prepared baking sheet.
4. **Bake** for about 20-25 minutes, stirring occasionally. Let cool, cut into bars and serve.

LUNCH

1. Oven Roasted Cauliflower

Servings: 7
Preparation time: 15 minutes
Cook time: 28 minutes
Ready in: 43 minutes

Nutrition Facts

Serving Size 109 g

Amount Per Serving

Calories 72	Calories from Fat 39

	% Daily Value*
Total Fat 4.3g	**7%**
Saturated Fat 1.3g	**7%**
Trans Fat 0.0g	
Cholesterol 4mg	**1%**
Sodium 80mg	**3%**
Total Carbohydrates 5.6g	**2%**
Dietary Fiber 2.4g	**9%**
Sugars 1.2g	
Protein 3.3g	

Vitamin A 2%	•	Vitamin C 105%
Calcium 8%	•	Iron 0%

Nutrition Grade C+
* Based on a 2000 calorie diet

Ingredients
- 2 tablespoons minced garlic
- 1 1/2 tablespoons olive oil
- 8 cups large cauliflower florets
- 1.5 oz. grated parmesan cheese
- 1/2 teaspoon sea salt
- 1/4 teaspoon ground black pepper

- 1 tablespoon chopped fresh parsley

Directions
1. **Preheat** the oven to 450 degrees F (220 degrees C). Grease a large casserole dish and set it aside.
2. **Place** olive oil, garlic, and cauliflower in a large re-sealable bag and shake to blend.
3. **Pour** into the prepared casserole dish, and season with salt and pepper to taste.
4. **Bake** for 25 minutes, stirring halfway through. Top with Parmesan cheese and parsley, and broil for 3 to 5 minutes, until golden brown.

2. Oven Roast Low-Cal Chicken

Servings: 5
Preparation time: 10 minutes
Cook time: 1 hour
Ready in: 1 hour and 10 minutes

Nutrition Facts

Serving Size 90 g

Amount Per Serving

Calories 101	Calories from Fat 14

	% Daily Value*
Total Fat 1.6g	2%
Cholesterol 39mg	13%
Sodium 829mg	35%
Total Carbohydrates 5.0g	2%
Sugars 2.7g	
Protein 15.1g	

Vitamin A 0%	•	Vitamin C 2%
Calcium 1%	•	Iron 3%

Nutrition Grade C+
* Based on a 2000 calorie diet

Ingredients
- 6 skinless, boneless chicken breast halves
- 2 tablespoons crushed garlic
- 1 1/2 tablespoons minced onion
- 1/2 teaspoon dried sage
- 1/2 teaspoon thyme

- 1/2 teaspoon rosemary
- 1/4 cup soy sauce
- 2 teaspoons raw honey

Directions
1. **Preheat** oven to 425 degrees F (220 degrees C).
2. **Place** chicken in a 9x13 inch baking dish and sprinkle with garlic, onion, sage, thyme, rosemary, soy sauce, and honey. Cover pan with foil.
3. **Bake** for 1 hour. Serve warm.

3. Crumbled Bacon and Shredded Brussels Sprouts

Servings: 5
Preparation time: 10 minutes
Cook time: 30 minutes
Ready in: 40 minutes

Nutrition Facts

Serving Size 81 g

Amount Per Serving

Calories 211   Calories from Fat 153

% Daily Value*

Total Fat 17.0g	**26%**
Saturated Fat 5.7g	**28%**
Trans Fat 0.0g	
Cholesterol 34mg	**11%**
Sodium 676mg	**28%**
Total Carbohydrates 5.4g	**2%**
Dietary Fiber 2.3g	**9%**
Sugars 1.3g	
Protein 10.5g	

Vitamin A 10%	Vitamin C 65%
Calcium 3%	Iron 7%

Nutrition Grade C-

* Based on a 2000 calorie diet

Ingredients
- 1/4 pound sliced bacon
- 1 1/2 tablespoons butter
- 1/4 cup pecan nuts
- 1/2 pound Brussels sprouts, cored and sliced
- 2 tablespoon green onions, minced

- 1/4 teaspoon sea salt
- 1/4 teaspoon ground black pepper

Directions

1. **Cook** bacon over medium-high heat until crisp. Take off bacon then crumble and set aside. Drain skillet, reserving 2 tablespoons grease.
2. **Melt** butter in with the reserved bacon grease over medium heat. Add pine nuts and cook until browned.
3. **Add** Brussels sprouts and green onions to the pan, and season with salt and pepper. Cook over medium heat until sprouts are wilted and tender for 10 to 15 minutes.
4. **Stir** in crumbled bacon before serving.

4. Indiana-Style Fried Cabbage

Servings: 7
Preparation time: 15 minutes
Cook time: 25 minutes
Ready in: 40 minutes

Nutrition Facts

Serving Size 100 g

Amount Per Serving

Calories 130	Calories from Fat 84

	% Daily Value*
Total Fat 9.3g	**14%**
Saturated Fat 3.8g	**19%**
Trans Fat 0.0g	
Cholesterol 24mg	**8%**
Sodium 408mg	**17%**
Total Carbohydrates 4.8g	**2%**
Dietary Fiber 1.8g	**7%**
Sugars 2.5g	
Protein 7.1g	

Vitamin A 9%	•	Vitamin C 51%
Calcium 3%	•	Iron 4%

Nutrition Grade B
* Based on a 2000 calorie diet

Ingredients

- 1/4 pound bacon, diced
- 1 1/2 tablespoons butter

- 1/2 small head cabbage, chopped
- 1/2 cup chopped celery
- 1/2 green bell pepper, chopped
- Sea salt and pepper to taste
- 1/2 cup sliced mushrooms
- 1/2 onion, chopped

Directions
1. **Cook** bacon until crisp over medium heat in a large deep skillet.
2. **Stir** in butter, cabbage, celery, green pepper, salt, pepper, mushrooms and onions.
3. **Steam** for 15- 20 minutes. Stir several times during the course of steaming.
4. **Place** in a dish and serve warm.

5. Lemon Roasted Tilapia

Servings: 5
Preparation time: 15 minutes
Cook time: 37 minutes
Ready in: 52 minutes

Nutrition Facts

Serving Size 213 g

Amount Per Serving

Calories 181   Calories from Fat 45

	% Daily Value*
Total Fat 5.0g	**8%**
Saturated Fat 1.1g	**6%**
Trans Fat 0.0g	
Cholesterol 69mg	**23%**
Sodium 53mg	**2%**
Total Carbohydrates 8.7g	**3%**
Dietary Fiber 1.3g	**5%**
Sugars 5.0g	
Protein 27.1g	

Vitamin A 2%	•	Vitamin C 43%
Calcium 4%	•	Iron 11%

Nutrition Grade C+

* Based on a 2000 calorie diet

Ingredients
- 5 (6 ounce) tilapia fillets
- 2 cloves roasted garlic, minced
- 1 tablespoon lemon pepper
- 1 tablespoon fresh parsley, chopped
- 2 medium lemons, sliced into rounds
- 1 onion, thinly sliced
- 1 1/2 tablespoons olive oil
- 1/2 cup fresh orange juice
- 1 1/2 tablespoons fresh lemon juice
- 2 teaspoons raw honey

Directions
1. **Preheat** the oven to 400 degrees F (200 degrees C).
2. **Mix** together the garlic, lemon pepper, and parsley in a small bowl. Arrange the slices from one of the lemons in a 9x13 inch baking dish.
3. **Add** onion slices over the oranges. Sprinkle with olive oil and half of the garlic mixture.
4. **Roast** for 25 minutes or until the onions are browned and tender. Remove dish from the oven and increase the temperature to 450 degrees F.
5. **Place** the tilapia fish at the center of the dish and move the onion and orange slices to the outer edge. Season fish with the remaining garlic mixture.
6. **Whisk** together the orange juice, lemon juice and honey in a small bowl and pour evenly over the tilapia.
7. **Bake** for 12-15 minutes. Transfer tilapia to a plate and discard roasted lemon slices.
8. **Serve** fillets with roasted onions and remaining fresh lemon slices.

6. Feta Bacon and Green Beans

Servings: 5
Preparation time: 10 minutes
Cook time: 18 minutes
Ready in: 28 minutes

Nutrition Facts

Serving Size 145 g

Amount Per Serving

Calories 122 — Calories from Fat 52

% Daily Value*

Total Fat 5.7g	**9%**
Saturated Fat 3.4g	**17%**
Trans Fat 0.0g	
Cholesterol 36mg	**12%**
Sodium 451mg	**19%**
Total Carbohydrates 7.8g	**3%**
Dietary Fiber 3.1g	**12%**
Sugars 2.3g	
Protein 9.7g	

Vitamin A 14%	•	Vitamin C 25%
Calcium 15%	•	Iron 6%

Nutrition Grade A-
* Based on a 2000 calorie diet

Ingredients

- 8 slices turkey bacon
- 1 (16 ounce) green beans, cut into 1.5-inch pieces
- 1 teaspoon chopped garlic
- 4 ounces crumbled feta cheese, divided
- 1 medium red onion, minced
- 1/8 teaspoon ground black pepper

Directions

1. **Cook** bacon in a skillet medium high heat until evenly brown but only slightly crisp. Drain bacon on paper towels. Leave about 3 tablespoons of bacon grease in the skillet and discard remaining grease. Crumble bacon, reserving 2 tablespoons for garnish, set aside.
2. **Steam** green beans for 10 minutes. Set aside.

3. **Sauté** garlic until lightly browned in the same skillet with the remaining bacon grease over medium-high heat.
4. **Add** the bacon, green beans, feta cheese, and onion; season with pepper. Cook for 2 minutes.
5. **Serve** topped with remaining feta cheese and crumbled bacon.

7. Spinach Torta

Servings: 3
Preparation time: 10 minutes
Cook time: 10 minutes
Ready in: 20 minutes

Nutrition Facts

Serving Size 168 g

Amount Per Serving

Calories 120	Calories from Fat 56

	% Daily Value*
Total Fat 6.3g	**10%**
Saturated Fat 2.1g	**10%**
Trans Fat 0.0g	
Cholesterol 67mg	**22%**
Sodium 447mg	**19%**
Total Carbohydrates 7.7g	**3%**
Dietary Fiber 2.6g	**10%**
Sugars 3.7g	
Protein 9.3g	

Vitamin A 215%	•	Vitamin C 53%
Calcium 12%	•	Iron 19%

Nutrition Grade A
* Based on a 2000 calorie diet

Ingredients
- 1 (12 oz.) packed spinach
- 1 egg
- 1/4 cup milk
- 1 tablespoon bacon bits
- 2 tablespoons Worcestershire sauce
- 1/2 teaspoon garlic powder
- 1 pinch red pepper flakes

Directions

1. **Boil** water in a deep skillet and steam spinach for 1 minute. Drain water and set aside.
2. **Whisk** egg, milk, garlic powder, Worcestershire sauce, pepper, and bacon bits together in a small bowl, then pour mixture into the skillet with spinach.
3. **Cook** over a medium-low heat; stirring frequently until most of the moisture is absorbed into the spinach. Serve warm.

8. Prosciutto and Swiss Cheese Stuffed Chicken

Servings: 6
Preparation time: 15 minutes
Cook time: 40 minutes
Ready in: 55 minutes

Nutrition Facts

Serving Size 319 g

Amount Per Serving

Calories 602   Calories from Fat 313

	% Daily Value*
Total Fat 34.8g	**54%**
Saturated Fat 19.1g	**96%**
Cholesterol 211mg	**70%**
Sodium 1434mg	**60%**
Total Carbohydrates 7.8g	**3%**
Sugars 0.9g	
Protein 56.1g	

Vitamin A 21%	•	Vitamin C 1%
Calcium 25%	•	Iron 9%

Nutrition Grade D

* Based on a 2000 calorie diet

Ingredients

- 6 skinless, boneless chicken breast halves , pounded flat
- 6 slices Swiss cheese
- 6 slices prosciutto
- 3 tablespoons bread crumbs
- 1 teaspoon paprika
- 6 tablespoons butter
- 1/2 cup dry white wine
- 1 teaspoon chicken bouillon granules

- 1 tablespoon cornstarch
- 1 cup heavy whipping cream
- 1 egg white

Directions

1. **Place** a cheese and prosciutto slice on each breast within 1/2 inch of the edges. Fold the edges of the chicken over the filling, and secure with toothpicks.
2. **Mix** the breadcrumbs and paprika in a small bowl. Coat chicken with egg white and rolled in breadcrumb mix.
3. **Melt** butter in a large skillet over medium-high heat, and cook the chicken until browned on all sides. Add the wine and bouillon. Reduce heat to low, cover, and simmer for 30 minutes, until chicken is no longer pink and juices run clear.
4. **Remove** the toothpicks, and transfer the breasts to a warm platter. Cut into halves.
5. **Blend** cornstarch with the cream in a small bowl, and whisk slowly into the skillet. Stir until thickened, and pour over the chicken. Serve warm.

9. Grilled Alaska Salmon with Oven Roasted Asparagus

Servings: 8
Preparation time: 4 hours
Cook time: 40 minutes
Ready in: 4 hours and 40 minutes

Nutrition Facts

Serving Size 199 g

Amount Per Serving

Calories 321	Calories from Fat 195

% Daily Value*

Total Fat 21.7g	**33%**
Saturated Fat 3.9g	**20%**
Trans Fat 0.0g	
Cholesterol 85mg	**28%**
Sodium 942mg	**39%**
Total Carbohydrates 6.6g	**2%**
Dietary Fiber 1.2g	**5%**
Sugars 4.4g	
Protein 24.8g	

Vitamin A 11%	Vitamin C 6%
Calcium 6%	Iron 9%

Nutrition Grade D+

* Based on a 2000 calorie diet

Ingredients

- 8 (4 ounce) salmon fillets
- 1/2 cup peanut oil
- 4 tablespoons soy sauce
- 4 tablespoons balsamic vinegar
- 4 tablespoons green onions, chopped
- 3 teaspoons brown sugar
- 2 cloves garlic, minced
- 1 1/2 teaspoons ground ginger
- 1 teaspoon crushed red pepper flakes
- 1 teaspoon sesame oil
- 1/2 teaspoon sea salt
- 1 tablespoon raw honey
- 1 (340 g) Asparagus bunch
- 1 tablespoon sea salt

- 2 tablespoon olive oil
- 1/2 teaspoon freshly ground black pepper

Directions

1. **Place** salmon filets in a medium, nonporous glass dish. In a separate medium bowl, combine the peanut oil, soy sauce, vinegar, green onions, brown sugar, garlic, ginger, red pepper flakes, sesame oil, honey and salt. Whisk together well, and pour over the fish. Cover and marinate the fish in the refrigerator for 4 to 6 hours.
2. **Prepare** an outdoor grill with coals about 5 inches from the grate, and lightly oil the grate.
3. **Grill** the fillets 5 inches from coals for 10 minutes per inch of thickness, measured at the thickest part, or until fish just flakes with a fork. Turn over halfway through cooking.
4. For the Side Dish: **Shake** to mix asparagus, salt, olive oil and pepper in big re-sealable bag.
5. **Rip off** a large piece of heavy duty aluminum foil, remove the asparagus from the plastic bag and wrap in the foil.
6. **Roast** in the oven at 350 degrees F for 30 minutes. Serve warm with the grilled salmon.

10. Parmesan Chicken Thigh

Servings: 4
Preparation time: 20 minutes
Cook time: 35 minutes
Ready in: 55 minutes

Nutrition Facts

Serving Size 152 g

Amount Per Serving

Calories 316	Calories from Fat 185

% Daily Value*

Total Fat 20.5g	**32%**
Saturated Fat 4.9g	**25%**
Trans Fat 0.0g	
Cholesterol 105mg	**35%**
Sodium 343mg	**14%**
Total Carbohydrates 6.5g	**2%**
Sugars 0.5g	
Protein 27.8g	

Vitamin A 4%	•	Vitamin C 0%
Calcium 16%	•	Iron 8%

Nutrition Grade D

* Based on a 2000 calorie diet

Ingredients

- 2 teaspoons crushed garlic
- 1/4 cup olive oil
- 1/4 cup Italian bread crumbs
- 1/4 cup grated Parmesan cheese
- 4 (4 oz.) skinless, boneless chicken thigh

Directions

1. **Preheat** oven to 425 degrees F (220 degrees C).
2. **Warm** the garlic and olive oil to blend the flavors. In a separate dish, combine the bread crumbs and Parmesan cheese.
3. **Dip** the chicken breasts in the olive oil and garlic mixture, then into the bread crumb mixture. Place in a shallow baking dish.
4. **Bake** in the preheated oven for 30 to 35 minutes, until no longer pink and juices run clear.

11. Mild Sausage, Peppers, and Onions

Servings: 6
Preparation time: 15 minutes
Cook time: 25 minutes
Ready in: 40 minutes

Nutrition Facts

Serving Size 205 g

Amount Per Serving

Calories 462	Calories from Fat 333

	% Daily Value*
Total Fat 37.0g	**57%**
Saturated Fat 11.0g	**55%**
Trans Fat 0.3g	
Cholesterol 95mg	**32%**
Sodium 852mg	**36%**
Total Carbohydrates 6.4g	**2%**
Dietary Fiber 1.7g	**7%**
Sugars 3.2g	
Protein 22.9g	

Vitamin A 31%	•	Vitamin C 108%
Calcium 3%	•	Iron 11%

Nutrition Grade C

* Based on a 2000 calorie diet

Ingredients

- 6 (4 ounce) Mild sausages
- 2 tablespoons olive oil
- 1 yellow onion, sliced
- 1/2 red onion, sliced
- 4 cloves garlic, minced
- 1 large red bell pepper, sliced
- 1 green bell pepper, sliced
- 1 teaspoon dried basil
- 1 teaspoon dried oregano
- 1/4 cup apple cider vinegar

Directions

1. **Place** the sausage in a large skillet over medium heat, and brown on all sides. Remove from skillet, and slice.

2. **Melt** butter in the skillet. Stir in the yellow onion, red onion, and garlic, and cook 2 to 3 minutes. Mix in red bell pepper and green bell pepper. Season with basil, and oregano.

3. **Stir** in cider vinegar. Continue to cook and stir until peppers and onions are tender.

4. **Return** sausage slices to skillet with the vegetables. Reduce heat to low, cover, and simmer 15 minutes, or until sausage is heated through.

12. Grapes, Pecan, Chicken Salad

Servings: 7
Preparation time: 20 minutes
Cook time: 20 minutes
Ready in: 40 minutes

Nutrition Facts

Serving Size 82 g

Amount Per Serving

Calories 157   Calories from Fat 88

% Daily Value*

Total Fat 9.8g	**15%**
Saturated Fat 1.6g	**8%**
Cholesterol 39mg	**13%**
Sodium 759mg	**32%**
Total Carbohydrates 6.3g	**2%**
Dietary Fiber 0.5g	**2%**
Sugars 2.2g	
Protein 11.6g	

Vitamin A 3%	•	Vitamin C 3%
Calcium 1%	•	Iron 5%

Nutrition Grade D+
* Based on a 2000 calorie diet

Ingredients

- 1 ½ (12 oz.) cups diced and chilled, cooked chicken meat
- 1/4 cup chopped celery
- 1/4 cup sliced, seedless red grapes
- 1/4 cup sliced pecans
- 1 tablespoon chopped fresh parsley
- 1/2 teaspoon sea salt
- 1/2 cup mayonnaise

- 1/8 cup heavy whipping cream

Directions
1. **Beat** whipping cream in medium bowl until soft peaks.
2. **Combine** meat, celery, grapes, almonds, parsley, salt, and mayonnaise with whipped cream. Chill.

13. Shrimp Caesar

Servings: 7
Preparation time: 20 minutes
Cook time: 20 minutes
Ready in: 40 minutes

Nutrition Facts

Serving Size 153 g

Amount Per Serving

Calories 217	Calories from Fat 99

% Daily Value*

Total Fat 10.9g	**17%**
Saturated Fat 4.1g	**21%**
Trans Fat 0.0g	
Cholesterol 158mg	**53%**
Sodium 720mg	**30%**
Total Carbohydrates 6.3g	**2%**
Dietary Fiber 1.5g	**6%**
Sugars 0.7g	
Protein 22.5g	

Vitamin A 9%	•	Vitamin C 39%
Calcium 20%	•	Iron 18%

Nutrition Grade B-
* Based on a 2000 calorie diet

Ingredients
- 3 tablespoons lemon juice, plus 4 lemon wedges for garnish
- 2 teaspoons Dijon mustard
- 3 anchovies, coarsely chopped
- 1 small clove garlic, coarsely chopped
- 2 tablespoons extra-virgin olive oil
- 1/2 (4 Oz) cup grated Asiago cheese, divided
- 1/2 teaspoon freshly ground pepper
- 8 cups chopped hearts of romaine, (about 2 hearts)
- 1 pound fresh shrimp, cooked

- 1 cup croutons, preferably whole-grain

Directions
1. **Place** lemon juice, mustard, anchovies (or anchovy paste) and garlic in a food processor; process until smooth. With the processor running, gradually add oil; process until creamy.
2. **Add** 1/4 cup Asiago cheese and pepper; pulse until combined.
3. **Combine** romaine, shrimp and croutons in a large bowl. Add the dressing and toss to coat.
4. **Divide** among 4 plates, top with the remaining 1/4 cup Asiago cheese and garnish with a lemon wedge.

14. Zesty Curried Chicken Salad

Servings: 8
Preparation time: 20 minutes
Cook time: 15 minutes
Ready in: 35 minutes

Nutrition Facts

Serving Size 133 g

Amount Per Serving

Calories 331   Calories from Fat 170

	% Daily Value*
Total Fat 18.9g	**29%**
Saturated Fat 4.5g	**23%**
Trans Fat 0.0g	
Cholesterol 89mg	**30%**
Sodium 624mg	**26%**
Total Carbohydrates 8.6g	**3%**
Sugars 3.3g	
Protein 30.4g	

Vitamin A 2%	•	Vitamin C 2%
Calcium 2%	•	Iron 7%

Nutrition Grade C+
* Based on a 2000 calorie diet

Ingredients
- 6 slices bacon
- 710 g diced cooked chicken breast meat
- 1/2 cup chopped celery
- 1 cup seedless grapes, halved

- 1/4 cup avocado
- 1 cup mayonnaise
- 1 teaspoon lemon juice
- 1/2 teaspoon curry powder
- 1/2 teaspoon Worcestershire sauce
- 2 tablespoons red onion, minced
- 1 teaspoon sea salt
- 1/2 teaspoon ground black pepper

Directions

1. **Cook** bacon in a large skillet over medium high heat until evenly browned. Drain on paper towels, crumble, and set aside.
2. **Combine** bacon, chicken, celery, grapes, and avocado in a large bowl.
3. **Whisk** together the mayonnaise, lemon juice, curry powder, Worcestershire sauce, onion, salt, and pepper in a small bowl.
4. **Pour** dressing over salad and toss well.

15. Spinach Salad with Bacon, Tomato, Avocado, and Ranch Dressing

Servings: 4
Ready in: 12 minutes

Nutrition Facts

Serving Size 192 g

Amount Per Serving

Calories 271	Calories from Fat 179

	% Daily Value*
Total Fat 19.9g	**31%**
Saturated Fat 5.3g	**26%**
Trans Fat 0.0g	
Cholesterol 93mg	**31%**
Sodium 895mg	**37%**
Total Carbohydrates 8.7g	**3%**
Dietary Fiber 4.2g	**17%**
Sugars 2.1g	
Protein 15.8g	

Vitamin A 116%	•	Vitamin C 42%
Calcium 8%	•	Iron 16%

Nutrition Grade A-
* Based on a 2000 calorie diet

Ingredients
- 16 ounces fresh baby spinach
- 1 cup grape tomatoes, halved, about 16
- 3 tablespoon red onion, sliced thin
- 3 hard-boiled eggs, sliced
- 1/2 pound bacon, cooked until crisp and crumbled
- 2 tablespoon almond, cooked
- 1 cup ranch dressing
- 2 cups avocados, mashed

Directions
1. **Mix** the ranch dressing with the avocado until smooth.
2. **Put** everything together in a large bowl and serve at once.

16. Andouille Jambalaya

Servings: 6
Preparation time: 15 minutes
Cook time: 40 minutes
Ready in: 55 minutes

Nutrition Facts

Serving Size 142 g

Amount Per Serving

Calories 127	Calories from Fat 68

% Daily Value*

Total Fat 7.6g	**12%**
Saturated Fat 2.0g	**10%**
Cholesterol 54mg	**18%**
Sodium 455mg	**19%**
Total Carbohydrates 5.5g	**2%**
Dietary Fiber 1.9g	**8%**
Sugars 2.4g	
Protein 9.8g	

Vitamin A 1%	•	Vitamin C 57%
Calcium 2%	•	Iron 9%

Nutrition Grade B-

* Based on a 2000 calorie diet

Ingredients

- 6 oz. Andouille sausage
- 1/8 cup olive oil
- 3/4 cup chopped onion
- 2 teaspoons crushed garlic
- 1/2 cup diced green peppers
- 1 cup diced fresh tomato
- 1/2 cup chicken broth
- 1/2 teaspoon dried thyme
- 1 medium head cauliflower
- 8 oz. medium shrimp
- 3/4 teaspoon sea salt
- 1/4 teaspoon ground black pepper
- 1/2 teaspoon Tabasco sauce

Directions

1. **Grease** a large pot with olive oil and on medium heat start browning sausage.
2. **Place** cauliflower through food processor to shred.
3. **Add** onion, garlic, and green pepper when sausage is lightly golden.
4. **Sauté** veggies until onion is translucent.
5. **Stir in** tomatoes, broth, thyme, and bring to simmer. Simmer for 20 minutes uncovered.
6. **Add** the shredded cauliflower and simmer for another 15 minutes until tender. Add shrimp and simmer for another 5 minutes and or so just long enough to cook the shrimp. Add salt and pepper and Tabasco to taste. Serve.

17. Creamy Chicken Soup

Servings: 6
Preparation time: 15 minutes
Cook time: 2 hours and 15 minutes
Ready in: 2 hours and 30 minutes

Nutrition Facts

Serving Size 261 g

Amount Per Serving

Calories 451   Calories from Fat 223

	% Daily Value*
Total Fat 24.8g	**38%**
Saturated Fat 11.6g	**58%**
Cholesterol 177mg	**59%**
Sodium 267mg	**11%**
Total Carbohydrates 7.6g	**3%**
Dietary Fiber 1.5g	**6%**
Sugars 2.6g	
Protein 47.6g	

Vitamin A 19%	Vitamin C 17%
Calcium 8%	Iron 17%

Nutrition Grade B-
* Based on a 2000 calorie diet

Ingredients

- 1 (2 to 3 pound) whole chicken
- 1 parsnip, sliced
- 1 turnip, quartered

105

- 2 mushrooms, quartered
- 2 stalks celery, quartered
- 1 leek, quartered
- 1 onion, quartered
- 3 sprigs fresh parsley
- 1 teaspoon chopped fresh dill
- 1 cup cream cheese
- Sea salt and pepper to taste

Directions

1. **Place** chicken, parsnip, turnip, mushroom, celery, leek, onion, parsley and dill in an 8 quart stock pot then cover with water and bring to a boil. Reduce the heat and simmer for 2 hours.
2. **Remove** the chicken from the soup, tear meat from bone, and set meat aside. Discard chicken bones, parsley and dill.
3. **Remove** vegetables from the stock pot. Using a food processor, puree vegetables. With processor running slowly add cream cheese.
4. **Return** puree vegetable in the stock pot and season with salt and pepper. Serve warm.

18. Southwestern Turkey Soup

Servings: 12
Preparation time: 15 minutes
Cook time: 30 minutes
Ready in: 45 minutes

Nutrition Facts

Serving Size 227 g

Amount Per Serving

Calories 132   Calories from Fat 62

	% Daily Value*
Total Fat 6.9g	**11%**
Saturated Fat 2.6g	**13%**
Trans Fat 0.0g	
Cholesterol 22mg	**7%**
Sodium 415mg	**17%**
Total Carbohydrates 7.6g	**3%**
Dietary Fiber 2.2g	**9%**
Sugars 3.8g	
Protein 10.5g	

Vitamin A 13%   •   Vitamin C 52%
Calcium 9%   •   Iron 15%

Nutrition Grade A-
* Based on a 2000 calorie diet

Ingredients

- 4 cups vegetable broth
- 1 1/2 cups shredded cooked turkey meat
- 3 1/2 cups whole tomatoes, peeled
- 2 medium roma tomatoes, chopped
- 2 cloves garlic, crushed
- 1 onion, chopped
- 1/2 chopped green chile peppers
- 1 tablespoon lime juice
- 1/2 teaspoon cayenne pepper
- 1/2 teaspoon ground cumin
- 1 teaspoon sea salt, or to taste
- 1/2 teaspoon ground black pepper, or to taste
- 1 avocado - peeled, pitted and diced
- 1/2 teaspoon dried parsley
- 1 cup shredded Monterey Jack cheese

Directions

1. **Pour** the vegetable broth into a large pot over medium heat. Add turkey, tomatoes, garlic, onion, green chile peppers, and lime juice; stir to combine.

2. **Season** with cayenne, cumin, salt, and pepper. Bring to a boil, then reduce heat, and simmer 15 to 20 minutes.

3. **Stir** in avocado and parsley, and simmer for another 15 to 20 minutes, until slightly thickened. Serve soup topped with shredded cheese.

19. Salmon Egg Salad

Servings: 8
Ready in: 10 minutes

Nutrition Facts

Serving Size 151 g

Amount Per Serving

Calories 247	Calories from Fat 152

	% Daily Value*
Total Fat 16.9g	**26%**
Saturated Fat 3.3g	**17%**
Trans Fat 0.0g	
Cholesterol 160mg	**53%**
Sodium 271mg	**11%**
Total Carbohydrates 8.0g	**3%**
Dietary Fiber 0.5g	**2%**
Sugars 2.5g	
Protein 15.8g	

Vitamin A 29%	•	Vitamin C 10%
Calcium 4%	•	Iron 5%

Nutrition Grade B

* Based on a 2000 calorie diet

Ingredients

- 14 -15 ounces canned salmon, flaked (I use two 7-Oz vacuums packed pouches)
- 6 hard-boiled eggs, peeled and chopped
- 1/2 cup chopped onion
- 1/2 cucumber, peeled, seeded and chopped
- 1 1/2 teaspoons Dijon mustard
- 1/2-3/4 cup mayonnaise

- 1/8 teaspoon black pepper
- 1/2-3/4 teaspoon dried tarragon (double if using fresh)
- 1/4 teaspoon paprika
- sea salt, to taste
- 1/2 cup shredded carrot
- 1/2 cup red radish, diced
- 2 tablespoons chopped Basil

Directions
1. **Place** all ingredients in a large clean bowl and mix well.
2. **Serve** in a room temperature or best if chilled for a few hours to allow flavors to blend.

20. Dilled Avocado Shrimp Salad

Servings: 10
Preparation time: 2 hours and 15 minutes
Cook time: 10 minutes
Ready in: 2 hours and 25 minutes

Nutrition Facts

Serving Size 171 g

Amount Per Serving

Calories 246　　　　Calories from Fat 98

	% Daily Value*
Total Fat 10.9g	**17%**
Saturated Fat 1.9g	**10%**
Trans Fat 0.0g	
Cholesterol 245mg	**82%**
Sodium 542mg	**23%**
Total Carbohydrates 10.3g	**3%**
Dietary Fiber 1.2g	**5%**
Sugars 2.1g	
Protein 26.5g	

Vitamin A 10%	•	Vitamin C 17%
Calcium 12%	•	Iron 5%

Nutrition Grade B
* Based on a 2000 calorie diet

Ingredients
- 2 1/2 pounds cooked shrimp - peeled and deveined
- 2 lemons, juiced
- 1 lime, juiced

- 2 stalks celery, chopped
- 3 green onions, chopped
- 1 tablespoon chopped fresh dill weed
- 1 cup mayonnaise
- 1/2 teaspoon sea salt
- 1/2 cup avocado
- ground black pepper to taste

Directions

1. **Chop** cooked shrimp into small pieces and place in a large bowl; squeeze lemon and lime juice over shrimp.
2. **Add** sliced avocado, celery, green onions, dill, mayonnaise, salt and pepper; mix well.
3. **Refrigerate** for 2 hours to allow flavors to combine; bring to room temperature for 15 minutes before serving.

21. Rosemary Roasted Turkey with Rhubarb Cranberry Sauce

Servings: 10
Preparation time: 30 minutes
Cook time: 5 hours
Ready in: 5 hours and 30 minutes

Nutrition Facts

Serving Size 646 g

Amount Per Serving

Calories 755	Calories from Fat 182

	% Daily Value*
Total Fat 20.2g	**31%**
Saturated Fat 2.2g	**11%**
Trans Fat 0.0g	
Cholesterol 340mg	**113%**
Sodium 1049mg	**44%**
Total Carbohydrates 10.1g	**3%**
Dietary Fiber 2.1g	**8%**
Sugars 1.9g	
Protein 112.6g	

Vitamin A 3%	•	Vitamin C 21%
Calcium 6%	•	Iron 43%

Nutrition Grade C-

* Based on a 2000 calorie diet

Ingredients

- 3/4 cup olive oil
- 3 tablespoons minced garlic
- 2 tablespoons chopped fresh rosemary
- 1 tablespoon chopped fresh basil
- 1 teaspoon marjoram, minced
- 1 teaspoon dried oregano, minced
- 1 teaspoon thyme, minced
- 1 teaspoon sage, minced
- 1 teaspoon ground black pepper
- sea salt to taste
- 12 pounds Fresh Whole Turkey
- 3 cups diced rhubarb (use unsweetened, frozen rhubarb if fresh is unavailable)
- 1 cup fresh cranberries

111

- 2 teaspoons minced or grated fresh ginger root
- 1/2 cup orange juice
- 3/4 cup water
- 4 tablespoons unprocessed brown sugar
- 1 tablespoon grated orange zest
- 1 cinnamon stick

Directions

1. **Preheat** oven to 325 degrees F (165 degrees C).
2. **Mix** the olive oil, garlic, rosemary, basil, oregano, sage, thyme, marjoram, black pepper and salt in a small bowl. Set aside.
3. **Wash** the turkey inside and out; pat dry. Remove any large fat deposits. Loosen the skin from the breast. This is done by slowly working your fingers between the breast and the skin. Work it loose to the end of the drumstick, being careful not to tear the skin.
4. **Spread** a generous amount of the rosemary mixture under the breast skin and down the thigh and leg. Rub the remainder of the rosemary mixture over the outside of the breast. Use toothpicks to seal skin over any exposed breast meat.
5. **Place** the turkey on a rack in a roasting pan. Add about 1/4 inch of water to the bottom of the pan. Roast in the preheated oven 3 to 4 hours, or until the internal temperature of the bird reaches 180 degrees F (80 degrees C).
6. *For the sauce:* **Place** rhubarb, cranberries, ginger, orange juice and zest, water and cinnamon stick in a large pot over medium heat, stirring to combine. Bring to a boil. Then reduce heat to medium-low and cover.
7. **Simmer** for 10 minutes or until rhubarb is tender and cranberries have popped.
8. **Stir** in brown sugar to taste and continue to simmer, uncovered, for 5 minutes. The sauce should be thick but still have a liquid consistency. Add more water, if necessary. Remove cinnamon stick and serve warm with the roasted turkey.

DINNER

1. Grilled Halibut Fillets

Servings: 3
Preparation time: 15 minutes
Cook time: 20 minutes
Ready in: 35 minutes

Nutrition Facts

Serving Size 285 g

Amount Per Serving

Calories 296	Calories from Fat 75

% Daily Value*

Total Fat 8.3g	**13%**
Saturated Fat 1.0g	**5%**
Trans Fat 0.0g	
Cholesterol 73mg	**24%**
Sodium 454mg	**19%**
Total Carbohydrates 2.5g	**1%**
Sugars 0.6g	
Protein 48.5g	

Vitamin A 16%	•	Vitamin C 8%	
Calcium 12%	•	Iron 13%	

Nutrition Grade C-

* Based on a 2000 calorie diet

Ingredients
- 1 teaspoon olive oil, plus extra amount for greasing
- 2 cloves garlic, finely chopped
- 1 medium shallot, finely chopped
- 1 tablespoon oyster sauce
- 1/2 cup apple cider vinegar
- 1 tablespoon low-sodium soy sauce
- 6 (4 ounce) fillets halibut, skin removed

113

- 1 teaspoon ginger oil
- 1/2 teaspoon red pepper flakes
- 1/4 teaspoon ground black pepper
- 2 tablespoons chopped fresh parsley

Directions
1. **Heat** olive oil in a saucepan over medium heat. Add garlic and shallot; cook until lightly browned.
2. **Stir** in the oyster sauce, cider vinegar, and soy sauce. Bring to boil and simmer until mixture is reduced by half. Set aside.
3. **Rub** fish fillets with ginger oil and sprinkle with red pepper flakes and black pepper.
4. **Preheat** an outdoor grill for high heat, and lightly oil grate with olive oil.
5. **Grill** fish for about 5 minutes per side, or just until cooked through.
6. **Pour** the prepared sauce over top. Sprinkle with parsley and serve.

2. Tuna Salad with Fresh Herbs

Servings: 4
Ready in: 10 minutes

Nutrition Facts

Serving Size 109 g

Amount Per Serving

Calories 172	Calories from Fat 86

	% Daily Value*
Total Fat 9.5g	**15%**
Saturated Fat 2.2g	**11%**
Cholesterol 138mg	**46%**
Sodium 156mg	**6%**
Total Carbohydrates 4.7g	**2%**
Dietary Fiber 0.7g	**3%**
Sugars 1.5g	
Protein 16.8g	

Vitamin A 13%	•	Vitamin C 12%
Calcium 10%	•	Iron 14%

Nutrition Grade A-
* Based on a 2000 calorie diet

Ingredients

- 6 ounce fresh tuna, shredded
- 1/4 cup chopped fresh dill weed
- 1/4 cup diced celery
- 1 tablespoon fresh lemon juice
- 2 tablespoons chopped fresh parsley
- 2 tablespoons thinly sliced chives
- 2 tablespoons plain low-fat yogurt
- 2 tablespoons light mayonnaise
- 1/2 teaspoon prepared Dijon-style mustard
- 3 hard-boiled eggs, chopped

Directions

1. **Combine** tuna with dill, celery, lemon juice, parsley, and chives in a medium bowl.
2. **Stir** together the yogurt, mayonnaise, and mustard in a small bowl until well blended.
3. **Add** mayonnaise mixture into the tuna mixture.
4. **Fold** in the eggs and toss well.
5. **Chill** before serving.

3. Cheddar Tilapia Fillets

Servings: 4
Preparation time: 10 minutes
Cook time: 10 minutes
Ready in: 20 minutes

Nutrition Facts

Serving Size 180 g

Amount Per Serving

Calories 286   Calories from Fat 140

	% Daily Value*
Total Fat 15.6g	**24%**
Saturated Fat 6.1g	**30%**
Trans Fat 0.0g	
Cholesterol 91mg	**30%**
Sodium 423mg	**18%**
Total Carbohydrates 5.0g	**2%**
Dietary Fiber 1.0g	**4%**
Protein 32.7g	

Vitamin A 17%	•	Vitamin C 4%
Calcium 18%	•	Iron 12%

Nutrition Grade C-
* Based on a 2000 calorie diet

Ingredients

- 1/4 cup whole wheat Panko breadcrumbs
- 3/4 cup grated sharp cheddar cheese
- 2 teaspoons paprika
- 2 cloves garlic, chopped
- 1 tablespoon chopped fresh parsley
- 1/2 teaspoon sea salt
- 1/4 teaspoon ground black pepper
- 4 (5 oz.) tilapia fillets
- 2 tablespoons olive oil

Directions

1. **Preheat** oven to 400 degrees F (200 degrees C). Line a baking sheet with aluminum foil.
2. **Combine** the breadcrumbs, cheese, paprika, garlic, parsley, salt, and pepper in a shallow dish.

3. **Drizzle** tilapia fillets with olive oil and dredge in the breadcrumb mixture.
4. **Place** coated fillets onto the prepared baking sheet.
5. **Bake** for 10 to 12 minutes or until the fish flakes easily with a fork.

4. Grilled Rosemary Citrus Swordfish

Servings: 4
Preparation time: 1 hour and 10 minutes
Cook time: 10 minutes
Ready in: 1 hour 20 minutes

Nutrition Facts

Serving Size 169 g

Amount Per Serving

Calories 224   Calories from Fat 86

	% Daily Value*
Total Fat 9.5g	**15%**
Saturated Fat 2.1g	**11%**
Trans Fat 0.0g	
Cholesterol 57mg	**19%**
Sodium 251mg	**10%**
Total Carbohydrates 3.2g	**1%**
Dietary Fiber 0.8g	**3%**
Sugars 0.5g	
Protein 29.2g	

Vitamin A 6%	•	Vitamin C 17%
Calcium 3%	•	Iron 11%

Nutrition Grade B+
* Based on a 2000 calorie diet

Ingredients
- 4 (4 ounce) swordfish steaks
- 1/4 teaspoon sea salt
- 1/4 teaspoon ground black pepper
- 3 cloves garlic, minced
- 2 teaspoons dried rosemary
- 1/2 cup apple cider vinegar
- 2 tablespoon thinly sliced scallions
- 1 tablespoon finely chopped parsley
- 1 teaspoon dried basil
- 2 tablespoons lime juice

- 1 tablespoon olive oil
- 4 slices lemon, for garnish

Directions

1. **Place** fish in a baking dish and season with salt and pepper. Combine garlic, rosemary, and apple cider vinegar in a small bowl. Pour mixture over fish, turning to coat.
2. **Cover**, and marinate in the fridge for at least 1 hour.
3. **Stir** together the scallions, parsley, basil, lime juice, olive oil, and remaining rosemary.
4. **Preheat** grill for medium heat.
5. **Grill** fish for 10 minutes, turning once, until fish is flakey.
6. **Pour** the prepared lime sauce on top of fish then garnish with lemon slices to serve.

5. Grilled Salmon Fillets

Servings: 6
Preparation time: 30 minutes
Cook time: 20 minutes
Ready in: 50 minutes

Nutrition Facts

Serving Size 361 g

Amount Per Serving

Calories 757   Calories from Fat 443

	% Daily Value*
Total Fat 49.2g	**76%**
Saturated Fat 9.4g	**47%**
Cholesterol 191mg	**64%**
Sodium 190mg	**8%**
Total Carbohydrates 8.4g	**3%**
Dietary Fiber 3.8g	**15%**
Sugars 1.0g	
Protein 68.0g	

Vitamin A 10%	•	Vitamin C 41%
Calcium 21%	•	Iron 62%

Nutrition Grade B+
* Based on a 2000 calorie diet

Ingredients

- 2 (2 pound) salmon fillets, skin removed
- 1/3 cup gluten-free soy sauce

- 1/3 cup olive oil
- 1 1/2 tablespoons rice vinegar
- 1 teaspoon garlic, minced
- 1 tablespoon fresh ginger, grated
- 1/4 cup green onions, chopped
- 1 cup fresh thyme, chopped
- 1/2 cup onions, chopped
- 1 fresh lemon, juiced
- 3 (12-inch) untreated cedar planks

Directions

1. **Soak** the cedar planks in warm water for at least 1 hour, or overnight.
2. **Place** the salmon fillets in a shallow dish. Stir together the soy sauce, olive oil, rice vinegar, garlic, ginger, and green onions in a small bowl.
3. **Pour** the marinade over the salmon fillets; turn once to coat evenly. Cover and marinate for at least 15 minutes or 1 hour.
4. **Mix** together the thyme, onions and lemon juice. Press mixture onto the top side of the fillets.
5. **Preheat** an outdoor grill for medium heat. Place the planks on the grill with the lid closed, for 3 minutes, or until they start to crackle and smoke.
6. **Arrange** the fillets, skin side down, onto the planks; spacing fillets 1 inch apart. Cover, and grill for about 20 minutes.
7. **Remove** planks from the grill. Place fillets onto plates and serve.

6. Spicy Meatball Nirvana

Servings: 6
Preparation time: 15 minutes
Cook time: 20 minutes
Ready in: 35 minutes

Nutrition Facts

Serving Size 115 g

Amount Per Serving

Calories 204	Calories from Fat 66

% Daily Value*

Total Fat 7.3g	**11%**
Saturated Fat 3.0g	**15%**
Trans Fat 0.1g	
Cholesterol 88mg	**29%**
Sodium 379mg	**16%**
Total Carbohydrates 8.4g	**3%**
Dietary Fiber 1.0g	**4%**
Sugars 2.1g	
Protein 23.4g	

Vitamin A 3%	•	Vitamin C 3%
Calcium 6%	•	Iron 15%

Nutrition Grade B
* Based on a 2000 calorie diet

Ingredients

- 1 pound extra lean ground beef
- 1/2 teaspoon sea salt
- 1 small onion, diced
- 1 clove garlic, finely chopped
- 1 1/2 teaspoons Italian seasoning
- 3/4 teaspoon crushed red pepper flakes
- 1 dash low-sodium organic hot sauce
- 1 1/2 tablespoons Worcestershire sauce
- 1 egg
- 1/4 cup grated Parmesan cheese
- 1/2 cup whole wheat bread crumbs

Directions

1. **Preheat** an oven to 400 degrees F (200 degrees C).
2. **Mix** all ingredients in a large bowl.

3. **Shape** into 1 1/2-inch meatballs then arrange on a baking sheet; spacing about 1 1/2-inches apart.
4. **Bake** for 20 to 25 minutes, until no longer pink in the center.

7. Classic Tourtiere

Servings: 6
Preparation time: 20 minutes
Cook time: 40 minutes
Ready in: 1 hour

Nutrition Facts

Serving Size 150 g

Amount Per Serving

Calories 280 | Calories from Fat 154

	% Daily Value*
Total Fat 17.1g	**26%**
Saturated Fat 2.5g	**12%**
Trans Fat 0.0g	
Cholesterol 61mg	**20%**
Sodium 537mg	**22%**
Total Carbohydrates 5.2g	**2%**
Dietary Fiber 1.2g	**5%**
Sugars 0.8g	
Protein 26.2g	

Vitamin A 1%	•	Vitamin C 4%
Calcium 1%	•	Iron 42%

Nutrition Grade C+
* Based on a 2000 calorie diet

Ingredients
- 1 pound lean ground pork
- 1/2 pound lean ground beef
- 1 1/2 teaspoons sea salt
- 1/4 teaspoon ground black pepper
- 1/2 teaspoon dried thyme, crushed
- 1/4 teaspoon ground rosemary
- 1/2 teaspoon ground cinnamon
- 1/8 teaspoon ground cloves
- 1 onion, diced
- 1 clove garlic, minced
- 1 egg
- 9 inch double whole wheat pie crust

Directions

1. **Preheat** oven to 425 degrees F (220 degrees C).
2. **Place** ground meat in a saucepan and season with salt, black pepper, thyme, rosemary, cinnamon, and cloves. Add the onion, garlic, and egg; mix well. Place the saucepan over medium heat.
3. Bring mixture to a boil; stirring occasionally. Reduce heat to low and simmer for 5 minutes until meat is cooked.
4. **Line** a 9-inch pie plate with bottom pie crust then add the meat mixture. Add the top crust and seal edges. Cut slits in top crust then cover edges with strips of aluminum foil.
5. **Bake** for 20 minutes. Remove foil, and then bake for 15 to 20 minutes more until golden brown.
6. **Let** cool, slice and serve.

8. Bacon and Bok Choy Stir Fry

Servings: 6
Preparation time: 15 minutes
Cook time: 15 minutes
Ready in: 30 minutes

Nutrition Facts

Serving Size 264 g

Amount Per Serving

Calories 221   Calories from Fat 135

	% Daily Value*
Total Fat 15.1g	**23%**
Saturated Fat 4.7g	**24%**
Trans Fat 0.0g	
Cholesterol 36mg	**12%**
Sodium 1033mg	**43%**
Total Carbohydrates 6.8g	**2%**
Dietary Fiber 2.4g	**9%**
Sugars 3.2g	
Protein 15.5g	

Vitamin A 139%	•	Vitamin C 130%
Calcium 17%	•	Iron 15%

Nutrition Grade A-
* Based on a 2000 calorie diet

Ingredients

- 6 slices bacon, chopped

- 1 teaspoon olive oil
- 1 small shallot, chopped
- 1 teaspoon dried cayenne pepper
- 2 cloves garlic, minced
- 2 pounds baby bok choy
- 1 medium celery stalk, chopped
- 1/2 cup sliced mushrooms
- 2 roma tomatoes, sliced
- 1/2 teaspoon sea salt
- 1/4 cup low-sodium chicken broth
- 1 green onion, chopped

Directions

1. **Cook** bacon in a large skillet over medium heat until browned on both sides. Remove bacon from pan and drain on paper towels. Leave 1 tablespoon of the grease in the skillet.
2. **Add** the olive oil, shallot, cayenne pepper, and garlic; cook, stirring occasionally until the shallot is translucent.
3. **Stir** in bok choy then cover and cook for 3 to 5 minutes. Add the celery, mushrooms, and tomatoes; season with salt and pour in the chicken broth.
4. **Stir** then simmer until bok choy is tender but still crunchy, about 2 minutes. Add the bacon and sprinkle with green onion. Serve warm.

9. Crispylicious Coconut Fish Sticks

Servings: 6
Preparation time: 15 minutes
Cook time: 20 minutes
Ready in: 35 minutes

Nutrition Facts

Serving Size 129 g

Amount Per Serving

Calories 285 — Calories from Fat 192

% **Daily Value***

Total Fat 21.4g	**33%**
Saturated Fat 16.5g	**83%**
Trans Fat 0.0g	
Cholesterol 82mg	**27%**
Sodium 252mg	**11%**
Total Carbohydrates 6.7g	**2%**
Dietary Fiber 3.6g	**15%**
Sugars 1.0g	
Protein 17.0g	

Vitamin A 5%	•	Vitamin C 4%
Calcium 2%	•	Iron 3%

Nutrition Grade D+

* Based on a 2000 calorie diet

Ingredients

- 2 eggs
- 1/2 cup coconut flour
- 1/2 teaspoon red pepper flakes
- 3 scallions, thinly sliced
- 1/4 cup dried basil
- 3 cloves garlic, finely chopped
- 1/2 teaspoon sea salt
- 1/4 teaspoon freshly ground black pepper
- 1/2 cup coconut oil
- 1 pound boneless cod fish, cut into 1-inch thick sticks

Directions

1. **Whisk** the eggs in a medium bowl.
2. **Mix** together the coconut flour, red pepper flakes, scallions, basil, garlic, salt, and black pepper in another bowl.

3. **Dip** fish sticks in egg, then flour mixture; coat well and place in a plate.
4. **Heat** coconut oil in a large skillet over medium high heat. Fry half of the fish sticks in coconut oil, 3 minutes on each side, or until golden brown.
5. **Drain** cooked fish sticks on paper towels. Work in batches if necessary, so you don't overcrowd the pan.

10. Red Chili Turkey Burger with Sautéed Okra

Servings: 6
Preparation time: 15 minutes
Cook time: 20 minutes
Ready in: 35 minutes

Nutrition Facts

Serving Size 171 g

Amount Per Serving

Calories 171   Calories from Fat 74

% **Daily Value***

Total Fat 8.2g	**13%**
Saturated Fat 2.1g	**10%**
Cholesterol 54mg	**18%**
Sodium 696mg	**29%**
Total Carbohydrates 9.8g	**3%**
Dietary Fiber 3.8g	**15%**
Sugars 3.7g	
Protein 16.7g	

Vitamin A 54%	•	Vitamin C 50%
Calcium 7%	•	Iron 14%

Nutrition Grade B+
* Based on a 2000 calorie diet

Ingredients
Turkey Burger:
- 1 cup red chilies, diced
- 1 pound lean ground turkey
- 1 cup parsley, finely chopped
- 1/2 cup onion, finely chopped
- 2 cloves garlic, finely chopped
- 1 teaspoon ground coriander
- 1 teaspoon sea salt

Sautéed Okra:

- 1/2 pound fresh okra, trimmed
- 1 tablespoon olive oil
- 1 large clove garlic, minced
- 1/2 teaspoon red pepper flakes
- 1 teaspoon sea salt
- 1 lemon, cut into wedges

Directions

1. **Combine** all turkey burger ingredients in a large bowl and shape into 6 patties. Grill the burgers for 6 minutes on each side. Transfer cooked patties onto a plate and set aside.
2. **Heat** olive oil in a large skillet over medium heat. Add the okra and sauté for about 4 minutes, stirring frequently.
3. **Stir** in the garlic and red pepper flakes and cook for another 2 minutes, until the garlic is golden brown. Season with salt.
4. **Add** the sautéed okra to the grilled burger patties and garnish with lemon wedges to serve.

11. Fried Chicken with Basil Cream

Servings: 4
Preparation time: 15 minutes
Cook time: 15 minutes
Ready in: 30 minutes

Nutrition Facts

Serving Size 428 g

Amount Per Serving

Calories 520	Calories from Fat 218

% Daily Value*

Total Fat 24.2g	**37%**
Saturated Fat 12.7g	**63%**
Trans Fat 0.0g	
Cholesterol 202mg	**67%**
Sodium 774mg	**32%**
Total Carbohydrates 9.6g	**3%**
Dietary Fiber 1.1g	**4%**
Sugars 2.6g	
Protein 59.8g	

Vitamin A 25%	•	Vitamin C 68%
Calcium 17%	•	Iron 6%

Nutrition Grade C

* Based on a 2000 calorie diet

Ingredients

- 3 tablespoons butter
- 1/4 cup milk
- 1/4 cup dried whole wheat bread crumbs
- 4 (9 oz.) skinless, boneless chicken breasts
- 1/2 cup low-sodium chicken broth
- 1 cup half and half
- 1/2 cup sliced roasted red peppers
- 1 cup sliced mushrooms
- 2 teaspoons dried basil
- 1/2 cup grated Parmesan cheese
- 1/8 teaspoon ground black pepper

Directions

1. **Dip** chicken in milk, then coat with bread crumbs.

2. **Heat** butter in a skillet over medium heat. Add the coated chicken and cook for 5 minutes each side or until juices run clear. Remove from pan and set aside.
3. **Pour** the chicken broth into skillet and bring to a boil over medium heat. Add the half and half, roasted red peppers, and mushrooms; bring to a boil, stirring frequently. Reduce heat.
4. **Stir** in basil, cheese, and black pepper; simmer until heated through.
5. **Pour** basil cream over chicken to serve.

12. Pork Tenderloin in Cranberry-Spinach Salad

Servings: 8
Preparation time: 20 minutes
Cook time: 20 minutes
Ready in: 40 minutes

Nutrition Facts

Serving Size 156 g

Amount Per Serving

Calories 228   Calories from Fat 119

	% Daily Value*
Total Fat 13.2g	**20%**
Saturated Fat 1.7g	**8%**
Trans Fat 0.0g	
Cholesterol 41mg	**14%**
Sodium 86mg	**4%**
Total Carbohydrates 9.7g	**3%**
Dietary Fiber 2.7g	**11%**
Sugars 5.1g	
Protein 19.7g	

Vitamin A 107%   •   Vitamin C 30%
Calcium 8%   •   Iron 16%

Nutrition Grade A
* Based on a 2000 calorie diet

Ingredients
- 1 pound pork tenderloin
- 1 cup cider vinegar
- 1/4 cup raw honey
- 1 teaspoon Dijon mustard
- 1 teaspoon dried marjoram, crushed
- 3 tablespoons toasted sesame seeds

- 2 cloves garlic, crushed and chopped
- 2 medium red onions, sliced
- 2 tablespoons olive oil
- 1 pound baby spinach leaves
- 3/4 cup dried cranberries
- 3/4 cup toasted walnuts

Directions

1. **Preheat** oven to 425 degrees F.
2. **Stir** together the 1/2 cup of cider vinegar, 1/8 cup of honey, mustard, and marjoram in a bowl.
3. **Place** pork in shallow pan and brush the vinegar mixture onto meat.
4. **Bake** for 20-25 minutes. Slice meat into bite-size pieces and place into a large bowl.
5. **Whisk** together the sesame seeds, remaining 1/8 cup of honey, garlic, onions, 1/2 cup cider vinegar and olive oil; pour mixture into the meat.
6. **Add** spinach, cranberries, and walnuts; toss well and serve.

13. Parmesan Crusted Chicken

Servings: 6
Preparation time: 20 minutes
Cook time: 45 minutes
Ready in: 1 hour and 5 minutes

Nutrition Facts

Serving Size 252 g

Amount Per Serving

Calories 397 — Calories from Fat 192

% Daily Value*

Total Fat 21.3g	**33%**
Saturated Fat 11.2g	**56%**
Trans Fat 0.0g	
Cholesterol 89mg	**30%**
Sodium 1173mg	**49%**
Total Carbohydrates 12.8g	**4%**
Dietary Fiber 1.1g	**5%**
Sugars 1.2g	
Protein 36.2g	

Vitamin A 7%	Vitamin C 1%
Calcium 27%	Iron 6%

Nutrition Grade D+

* Based on a 2000 calorie diet

Ingredients

- 6 skinless, boneless chicken breasts
- 1 teaspoon sea salt
- 1/2 teaspoon ground black pepper
- 1/2 cup sliced cremini mushrooms
- 1/4 cup chopped cilantro
- 6 slices Parmesan cheese
- 1/3 cup apple cider vinegar
- 1 (10.75 ounce) can condensed cream of mushroom soup
- 1/4 cup sour cream
- 3/4 cup whole wheat Panko breadcrumbs
- 1/8 teaspoon dried parsley
- 3 cloves garlic, finely chopped
- 1/2 cup low-fat butter, melted

Directions

1. **Preheat** oven to 325 degrees F (165 degrees C).
2. **Season** chicken with salt and pepper then place it in a 9x13 inch baking dish. Cover each chicken breast with mushrooms, cilantro, and a slice of cheese.
3. **Combine** the cider vinegar, mushroom soup, and sour cream, and pour mixture over chicken.
4. **Stir** dried parsley, breadcrumbs, and garlic in butter, and sprinkle them on top of chicken.
5. **Bake** for 45 minutes, or until chicken is cooked through.

14. Golden Lemon Chicken Tenders

Servings: 5
Preparation time: 15 minutes
Cook time: 25 minutes
Ready in: 40 minutes

Nutrition Facts

Serving Size 170 g

Amount Per Serving

Calories 313   Calories from Fat 102

	% Daily Value*
Total Fat 11.4g	**18%**
Saturated Fat 3.7g	**19%**
Trans Fat 0.0g	
Cholesterol 159mg	**53%**
Sodium 552mg	**23%**
Total Carbohydrates 13.7g	**5%**
Dietary Fiber 1.6g	**6%**
Sugars 3.1g	
Protein 35.7g	

Vitamin A 6%	•	Vitamin C 19%
Calcium 11%	•	Iron 15%

Nutrition Grade B

* Based on a 2000 calorie diet

Ingredients

- 1/2 teaspoon paprika
- 1/2 teaspoon sea salt
- 1/4 teaspoon ground black pepper
- 3 (6 oz.) boneless, skinless chicken breasts, cut into 2-inch pieces

- 3/4 cup Italian seasoned whole wheat bread crumbs
- 1/4 cup grated parmesan cheese
- 2 eggs, slightly beaten
- 1/2 cup fresh lemon juice
- 1/4 cup stevia
- 1 1/2 teaspoons curry powder

Directions

1. **Preheat** oven to 400 degrees F (200 degrees C). Line a 15x10 inch baking sheet with aluminum foil.
2. **Season** chicken with paprika, salt, and pepper. Combine the breadcrumbs and cheese in a bowl.
3. **Dip** pieces in egg, and then dredge in the breadcrumb mixture. Arrange chicken pieces in a single layer in the prepared baking sheet.
4. **Bake** for 15 minutes, turning once.
5. **Place** the lemon juice, stevia, and curry powder a small saucepan over medium-low heat. Cook for 5 minutes; stirring often. Drizzle lemon sauce over chicken.
6. **Return** chicken to oven, and bake for additional 5 minutes.

15. Beef Jambalaya with Cauliflower Rice

Servings: 5
Preparation time: 10 minutes
Cook time: 25 minutes
Ready in: 35 minutes

Nutrition Facts

Serving Size 264 g

Amount Per Serving

Calories 225   Calories from Fat 92

% Daily Value*

Total Fat 10.2g	**16%**
Saturated Fat 2.4g	**12%**
Cholesterol 61mg	**20%**
Sodium 444mg	**19%**
Total Carbohydrates 10.9g	**4%**
Dietary Fiber 3.6g	**14%**
Sugars 6.1g	
Protein 23.2g	

Vitamin A 20%   •   Vitamin C 119%
Calcium 2%   •   Iron 81%

Nutrition Grade A

* Based on a 2000 calorie diet

Ingredients

- 2 tablespoon olive oil
- 3/4 pound lean ground beef
- 2 garlic cloves, minced
- 1 onion, chopped
- 1 green bell pepper, diced
- 1 head cauliflower, riced
- 3/4 cup organic tomato sauce
- 1 3/4 cup diced tomatoes
- 1 teaspoon dried basil
- 1/2 teaspoon dried thyme
- 1/2 teaspoon red pepper flakes
- 1/2 teaspoon sea salt
- 1/4 teaspoon ground black pepper

Directions

1. **Heat** olive oil in a skillet over medium-high heat. Add ground beef and cook until brown.

2. **Stir** in garlic and sauté until lightly browned. Add the onion and green bell pepper. Cover and let cook for about 5 minutes.

3. **Add** tomato sauce, diced tomatoes, and spices; blend well. Add the cauliflower rice and season with salt and pepper.

4. **Simmer** covered for 15 minutes, or until cauliflower is tender. Serve warm.

16. Honey Mustard Salmon Steaks

Servings: 4
Preparation time: 15 minutes
Cook time: 20 minutes
Ready in: 35 minutes

Nutrition Facts

Serving Size 209 g

Amount Per Serving

Calories 448   Calories from Fat 238

	% Daily Value*
Total Fat 26.4g	**41%**
Saturated Fat 5.0g	**25%**
Trans Fat 0.0g	
Cholesterol 111mg	**37%**
Sodium 576mg	**24%**
Total Carbohydrates 13.0g	**4%**
Sugars 9.7g	
Protein 38.3g	

Vitamin A 3%	•	Vitamin C 12%
Calcium 4%	•	Iron 5%

Nutrition Grade B-
* Based on a 2000 calorie diet

Ingredients

- 1/4 cup light mayonnaise
- 3 tablespoons Dijon mustard
- 2 tablespoons raw honey
- 1 teaspoon lemon juice
- 4 (6 ounce) salmon steaks

- 1/2 teaspoon sea salt
- 1/2 teaspoon ground black pepper

Directions
1. **Preheat** oven to 325 degrees F (165 degrees C).
2. **Stir** together the mayonnaise, mustard, honey, and lemon juice in a small bowl.
3. **Spread** the mixture over the salmon steaks then sprinkle with salt and pepper.
4. **Arrange** steaks in a medium baking dish.
5. **Bake** for 20 minutes or until fish easily flakes with a fork.

17. Roasted Pork Tenderloin with Blueberry Sauce

Servings: 4
Preparation time: 10 minutes
Cook time: 35 minutes
Ready in: 45 minutes

Nutrition Facts

Serving Size 191 g

Amount Per Serving

Calories 225   Calories from Fat 54

	% Daily Value*
Total Fat 6.0g	9%
Saturated Fat 1.6g	8%
Trans Fat 0.0g	
Cholesterol 83mg	28%
Sodium 301mg	13%
Total Carbohydrates 11.0g	4%
Dietary Fiber 1.5g	6%
Sugars 7.4g	
Protein 30.3g	

Vitamin A 1%	•	Vitamin C 9%
Calcium 2%	•	Iron 10%

Nutrition Grade A-

* Based on a 2000 calorie diet

Ingredients
- 1/2 teaspoon dried rosemary, crushed
- 1/2 teaspoon sea salt
- 1/2 teaspoon freshly ground black pepper
- 1/4 teaspoon garlic powder

- 1/4 teaspoon dry mustard powder
- 1/8 teaspoon celery seed
- 1/8 teaspoon dried parsley
- 1/8 teaspoon red pepper flakes
- 1-1/4 pound pork tenderloin

Blueberry sauce:
- 1 small red onion, diced
- 1-1/2 cups frozen blueberries, thawed
- 1/4 cup apple cider vinegar
- 1 tablespoon pure maple syrup
- 1/2 teaspoon freshly ground black pepper
- 1/2 tablespoon olive oil

Directions
1. **Preheat** oven to 400 degrees F.
2. **Mix** together the rosemary, salt, black pepper, garlic powder, mustard, celery seed, parsley, and red pepper flakes in a small bowl and rub onto the pork.
3. **Place** seasoned pork in a roasting pan, and roast in the preheated oven for 25 minutes (or until internal temperature reaches 155° F). Remove pork to a serving platter.
4. **Heat** olive oil in a small saucepan over medium-high heat. Add the onion and sauté for about 5 minutes, or until soft.
5. **Stir** the remaining sauce ingredients into the saucepan, and cook for another 5 minutes, or until sauce is thickened. Pour sauce over roasted pork to serve.

18. Peach Sauce over Pork Chops

Servings: 4
Preparation time: 10 minutes
Cook time: 25 minutes
Ready in: 35 minutes

Nutrition Facts

Serving Size 206 g

Amount Per Serving

Calories 241 — Calories from Fat 73

% Daily Value*

Total Fat 8.1g	**12%**
Saturated Fat 1.9g	**10%**
Trans Fat 0.0g	
Cholesterol 83mg	**28%**
Sodium 391mg	**16%**
Total Carbohydrates 11.3g	**4%**
Dietary Fiber 1.8g	**7%**
Sugars 8.7g	
Protein 30.9g	

Vitamin A 8% • Vitamin C 13%
Calcium 3% • Iron 12%

Nutrition Grade A-
* Based on a 2000 calorie diet

Ingredients

- 2 fresh peaches, peeled, cored, and diced
- 1/4 cup water
- 1 tablespoons raw honey
- 2 tablespoons Dijon mustard
- 2 teaspoons curry powder
- 1/2 teaspoon ground cinnamon
- 1 teaspoon ground ginger
- 1/2 teaspoon sea salt
- 1/4 teaspoon ground black pepper
- 1 tablespoon olive oil
- 4 (1/4-pound) boneless pork chops
- 2 green onions, chopped
- 2 tablespoons chopped fresh parsley

Directions

1. **Place** the peaches, water, and honey in a small saucepan over medium-high heat. Cook for 8 to minutes, or until tender.

2. **Puree** the peach mixture in blender until smooth then pour into a bowl. Add mustard and curry powder to the peach mixture; stir thoroughly.

3. **Sprinkle** pork chops with cinnamon, ginger, salt, and pepper.

4. **Heat** the olive oil in a skillet over medium heat. Add the seasoned pork chops and cook for 4 minutes each side.

5. **Pour** the peach mixture over the pork chops; simmer until heated through.

6. **Sprinkle** parsley and green onions over the top and serve.

19. Stir-Fried Shrimp 'N Broccoli

Servings: 5
Preparation time: 12 minutes
Cook time: 12 minutes
Ready in: 24 minutes

Nutrition Facts

Serving Size 233 g

Amount Per Serving

Calories 214	Calories from Fat 91

	% Daily Value*
Total Fat 10.1g	**16%**
Saturated Fat 1.3g	**7%**
Cholesterol 178mg	**59%**
Sodium 585mg	**24%**
Total Carbohydrates 10.2g	**3%**
Dietary Fiber 1.9g	**7%**
Sugars 2.6g	
Protein 22.9g	

Vitamin A 7%	•	Vitamin C 58%
Calcium 5%	•	Iron 25%

Nutrition Grade B

* Based on a 2000 calorie diet

Ingredients

- 3 tablespoon extra-virgin olive oil
- 2 cloves garlic, minced
- 4 green onions, chopped

- 2 tablespoon fresh ginger, minced
- 2 cups broccoli florets
- 2 cups sliced mushrooms
- 1lb. raw medium shrimp, peeled and deveined
- 1 cup low-sodium vegetable broth, mixed with 2 tablespoons cornstarch
- 2 teaspoons low-sodium soy sauce
- 3/4 teaspoon raw honey
- 1/4 teaspoon sea salt
- 1/4 teaspoon ground black pepper

Directions

1. **Heat** olive oil in a large skillet over high heat. Add the garlic, green onions, and ginger; stir and cook until garlic is lightly browned.
2. **Stir** in broccoli and mushrooms, and cook for 3 minutes until tender.
3. **Add** shrimp, cook for 3 minutes, stirring frequently until they turn pink. Pour in vegetable broth, soy sauce and honey.
4. **Cover** and simmer for 1 minute, until thickened. Stir and season with salt and pepper.

20. Tofu and Veggie Stir-Fry

Servings: 6
Preparation time: 15 minutes
Cook time: 20 minutes
Ready in: 35 minutes

Nutrition Facts

Serving Size 216 g

Amount Per Serving

Calories 162   Calories from Fat 101

	% Daily Value*
Total Fat 11.2g	**17%**
Saturated Fat 1.6g	**8%**
Trans Fat 0.0g	
Cholesterol 0mg	**0%**
Sodium 872mg	**36%**
Total Carbohydrates 10.9g	**4%**
Dietary Fiber 2.5g	**10%**
Sugars 2.9g	
Protein 7.9g	

Vitamin A 75%	•	Vitamin C 98%
Calcium 12%	•	Iron 9%

Nutrition Grade A

* Based on a 2000 calorie diet

Ingredients

- 1 tablespoon cornstarch
- 2 tablespoons soy sauce
- 2 1/2 tablespoons water
- 1/4 cup extra-virgin olive oil, divided
- 2 cloves garlic, crushed
- 2 teaspoons chopped fresh ginger root, divided
- 1 14-ounce package soft tofu, drained and cut into 1-inch cubes
- 1 small head broccoli, cut into florets
- 1 cup bean sprouts
- 3/4 cup julienned carrots
- 1/2 cup halved green beans
- 1/4 cup chopped onion
- 1/2 tablespoon sea salt

Directions

1. **Stir** together the cornstarch, soy sauce, and water in a small bowl. Set aside.
2. **Heat** olive oil in a large skillet over medium heat. Add the garlic and 1 teaspoon ginger, cook until garlic is lightly brown.
3. **Add** tofu and vegetables, cook for 2 minutes, stirring frequently. Pour in the cornstarch mixture into skillet.
4. **Mix** in onion, salt, and remaining 1 teaspoon ginger. Cook until vegetables are tender but still crisp.
5. **Serve** warm.

21. Coconut Chicken Curry

Servings: 8
Preparation time: 10 minutes
Cook time: 40 minutes
Ready in: 50 minutes

Nutrition Facts

Serving Size 229 g

Amount Per Serving

Calories 241   Calories from Fat 93

	% Daily Value*
Total Fat 10.3g	**16%**
Saturated Fat 3.3g	**16%**
Trans Fat 0.0g	
Cholesterol 76mg	**25%**
Sodium 491mg	**20%**
Total Carbohydrates 11.0g	**4%**
Dietary Fiber 1.7g	**7%**
Sugars 8.0g	
Protein 25.8g	

Vitamin A 52%	•	Vitamin C 7%
Calcium 13%	•	Iron 12%

Nutrition Grade B
* Based on a 2000 calorie diet

Ingredients

- 1 1/2 pounds boneless skinless chicken breasts, cut into 1/2-inch chunks
- 1 teaspoon sea salt
- 1 teaspoon ground black pepper
- 2 tablespoons curry powder

- 1 1/2 tablespoons olive oil
- 2 cloves garlic, crushed
- 1/2 onion, thinly sliced
- 1 cup diced carrots
- 1/2 cup chopped celery
- 1 3/4 cup pure coconut milk
- 1 3/4 cup can stewed, diced tomatoes
- 1 cup tomato sauce
- 2 tablespoons raw honey

Directions

1. **Place** chicken chunks in a bowl and season with salt, pepper, and curry powder.
2. **Heat** olive oil in a large skillet over medium-high heat.
3. **Sauté** garlic and onions in olive oil for 1 minute. Reduce heat to medium.
4. **Add** seasoned chicken and cook for 7 to 10 minutes or until chicken is no longer pink in the center and juices run clear. Add carrots and celery, simmer until tender.
5. **Stir** in coconut milk, tomatoes, tomato sauce, and honey. Cover and simmer for 30 minutes; stirring occasionally.
6. **Serve** warm.

DESSERT and SNACK

1. Heavenly Bacon

Servings: 6
Preparation time: 15 minutes
Cook time: 10 minutes
Ready in: 25 minutes

Nutrition Facts

Serving Size 213 g

Amount Per Serving

Calories 171	Calories from Fat 171

	% Daily Value*
Total Fat 68.2g	**105%**
Saturated Fat 7.2g	**36%**
Trans Fat 0.0g	
Cholesterol 35mg	**12%**
Sodium 425mg	**18%**
Total Carbohydrates 6.0g	**2%**
Dietary Fiber 1.2g	**5%**
Sugars 4.1g	
Protein 5.8g	

Vitamin A 5%	•	Vitamin C 0%
Calcium 1%	•	Iron 3%

Nutrition Grade D

* Based on a 2000 calorie diet

Ingredients
- 6 strips cooked bacon
- 4 tablespoons unsweetened cocoa powder
- 6 tablespoons stevia
- 4 tablespoon butter

Directions

1. **Place** cocoa, butter, and stevia in a bowl and microwave for 30-45 seconds on high heat. Stir after 30 seconds.
2. **Dip** bacon in the chocolate mixture to coat. Dry on cooling racks over parchment paper to catch drips. Best serve with low carb shakes.

2. Vanilla Almond Milkshake

Servings: 1
Ready in: 20 minutes

Nutrition Facts

Serving Size 310 g

Amount Per Serving

Calories 123	Calories from Fat 68

	% Daily Value*
Total Fat 7.5g	**12%**
Trans Fat 0.0g	
Cholesterol 0mg	**0%**
Sodium 451mg	**19%**
Total Carbohydrates 7.8g	**3%**
Dietary Fiber 3.0g	**12%**
Sugars 0.8g	
Protein 3.0g	

Vitamin A 0%	•	Vitamin C 0%
Calcium 0%	•	Iron 0%

Nutrition Grade D
* Based on a 2000 calorie diet

Ingredients

- 3 cups unsweetened almond milk
- 1 1/2 teaspoons pure vanilla extract
- 2 packets stevia

Directions

1. **Combine** 1 1/2 cups of almond milk, vanilla, and stevia.
2. **Pour** mixture into an ice cube tray and place in the freezer until completely firmed.
3. **Blend** frozen almond milk mixture in a blender along with the remaining 1 1/2 cup of almond milk until desired creaminess is achieved.

3. Guilt-Free Lemon Mousse

Servings: 8
Preparation time: 2 hours and 10 minutes
Cook time: 1 minute
Ready in: 2 hours and 11 minutes

Nutrition Facts

Serving Size 87 g

Amount Per Serving

Calories 203　　　　　Calories from Fat 171

	% Daily Value*
Total Fat 19.0g	**29%**
Saturated Fat 10.5g	**53%**
Trans Fat 0.0g	
Cholesterol 267mg	**89%**
Sodium 102mg	**4%**
Total Carbohydrates 8.0g	**3%**
Sugars 0.5g	
Protein 6.3g	

Vitamin A 12%	•	Vitamin C 7%	
Calcium 4%	•	Iron 3%	

Nutrition Grade D+

* Based on a 2000 calorie diet

Ingredients

- 1/2 cup low-fat butter
- 9 egg yolks
- 4 tablespoons lemon juice
- 2 teaspoons grated lemon zest
- 1/4 cup stevia
- 4 egg whites
- 1 teaspoon pure vanilla extract
- 1 1/2 cups heavy cream

Directions

1. **Melt** butter in a saucepan over low heat.
2. **Remove** from heat immediately, and then whisk in yolks one at a time.
3. **Beat** in lemon juice, zest, and 2 tablespoons of stevia. Chill the mixture.

Beat together the egg whites, vanilla extract, cream and the remaining stevia until smooth in a bowl.

Fold egg white mixture into the chilled egg yolk mixture.

Chill for at least 2 hours before serving.

i Seed Chocolate Brownies

Servings: 12
Preparation time: 35 minutes
Cook time: 35-50 minutes
Ready in: 1 hour and 10 minutes

Nutrition Facts

Serving Size 69 g

Amount Per Serving

Calories 165   Calories from Fat 131

	% Daily Value*
Total Fat 14.5g	**22%**
Saturated Fat 8.0g	**40%**
Trans Fat 0.0g	
Cholesterol 102mg	**34%**
Sodium 241mg	**10%**
Total Carbohydrates 8.1g	**3%**
Dietary Fiber 3.6g	**15%**
Protein 4.8g	

Vitamin A 9%	•	Vitamin C 0%
Calcium 5%	•	Iron 8%

Nutrition Grade D

* Based on a 2000 calorie diet

Ingredients

- 1 tablespoon chia seeds
- 1/2 cup water
- 1/4 cup almond flour
- 1/4 cup coconut flour
- 4 large eggs
- 3/4 cup unsweetened cocoa powder
- 1 stick butter, melted
- 2 teaspoons pure vanilla extract
- 1/2 teaspoon baking soda
- 1 teaspoon ground cinnamon
- 12 packets stevia

- 1/2 teaspoon organic sea salt
- 4 ounces cream cheese, melted
- coconut oil for greasing

Directions

1. **Grease** an 8x8 inch baking pan with coconut oil.
2. **Mix** 1 tablespoon chia seeds and water in a bowl. Let sit for 20 minutes, stirring every 10 minutes.
3. **Whisk** together the prepared chia gel, almond flour, and coconut flour. Add eggs, cocoa, butter, vanilla, baking soda, cinnamon, stevia, and salt; whisk to combine.
4. **Pour** the batter in the prepared baking pan and drop dollops of cream cheese onto batter. Gently swirl cream cheese onto the batter with a knife.
5. **Bake** for 35-50 minutes, or until toothpick inserted in the center of the brownie comes out clean.
6. **Let** cool and serve.

5. No Crust Raspberry Cheesecake

Servings: 8
Preparation time: 15 minutes
Cook time: 40 minutes
Ready in: 55 minutes

Nutrition Facts

Serving Size 75 g

Amount Per Serving

Calories 156   Calories from Fat 131

	% Daily Value*
Total Fat 14.5g	**22%**
Saturated Fat 8.8g	**44%**
Trans Fat 0.0g	
Cholesterol 85mg	**28%**
Sodium 103mg	**4%**
Total Carbohydrates 9.4g	**3%**
Protein 3.8g	

Vitamin A 11%	•	Vitamin C 0%
Calcium 4%	•	Iron 3%

Nutrition Grade D-

* Based on a 2000 calorie diet

Ingredients

- 8 oz. cream cheese, softened
- 1/3 cup stevia
- 1/2 teaspoon ground cinnamon
- 1/2 teaspoon pure vanilla extract
- 1 egg
- 3/4 cup whipping cream
- 1 cup halved raspberries

Directions

1. **Preheat** oven to 350 degrees.
2. **Mix** cream cheese, stevia, cinnamon, and vanilla in a large bowl. Beat well.
3. **Add** the egg and beat again. Pour batter in an 8 inch pie-plate.
4. **Bake** for 40- 45 minutes or until a toothpick inserted into the center comes out clean. Let cool.
5. **Spread** whipping cream on top and garnish with raspberries.

6. Light Choco Mousse

Servings: 10
Ready in: 15 minutes

Nutrition Facts

Serving Size 73 g

Amount Per Serving

Calories 132   Calories from Fat 81

	% Daily Value*
Total Fat 9.0g	**14%**
Saturated Fat 4.6g	**23%**
Trans Fat 0.0g	
Cholesterol 27mg	**9%**
Sodium 87mg	**4%**
Total Carbohydrates 12.9g	**4%**
Dietary Fiber 0.7g	**3%**
Sugars 2.4g	
Protein 6.7g	

Vitamin A 6%	•	Vitamin C 0%
Calcium 15%	•	Iron 3%

Nutrition Grade D+

* Based on a 2000 calorie diet

Ingredients
- 2 cups ricotta cheese
- 1/4 cup cream cheese, preferably whipped or softened
- 1/4 cup heavy whipping cream
- 1/3 cup stevia
- 2 tablespoons cocoa powder
- 2 tablespoon pure chocolate syrup
- 1 teaspoon pure vanilla extract
- 1/2 teaspoon ground cinnamon
- 1/4 cup chopped toasted pecans

Directions
1. **Process** ricotta, cream cheese and whipping cream with a hand mixer in a shallow bowl for 1-2 minutes, until smooth.
2. **Add** stevia, cocoa, chocolate syrup, vanilla, and cinnamon. Process until smooth and creamy.
3. **Spoon** into dessert cups and garnish with pecan nuts. Chill before serving.

7. Fresh Fruit Salad with Lemon Coconut Cream

Servings: 6
Ready in: 20 minutes

Nutrition Facts

Serving Size 115 g

Amount Per Serving

Calories 165 — Calories from Fat 109

	% Daily Value*
Total Fat 12.2g	**19%**
Saturated Fat 4.8g	**24%**
Trans Fat 0.0g	
Cholesterol 0mg	**0%**
Sodium 25mg	**1%**
Total Carbohydrates 11.8g	**4%**
Dietary Fiber 4.5g	**18%**
Sugars 6.9g	
Protein 4.3g	

Vitamin A 3%	•	Vitamin C 20%
Calcium 8%	•	Iron 7%

Nutrition Grade B+
* Based on a 2000 calorie diet

Ingredients

- 1 peach, pitted and sliced
- 1 cup sliced raspberries
- 1 cup fresh blueberries
- 3/4 cup chopped hazelnuts
- 2 tablespoons freshly squeezed lemon juice
- 1/2 cup coconut cream
- 1 cup plain soy milk
- 1/2 teaspoon ground cinnamon
- 2 tablespoons ground flax seeds

Directions

1. **Combine** peach, raspberries, blueberries, and hazelnuts in a large salad bowl.
2. **Stir** together lemon juice, coconut cream, soy milk, and cinnamon then pour over salad.
3. **Sprinkle** with ground flax seeds and gently toss to coat.
4. **Chill** and serve.

8. Low Carb Strawberry Cobbler

Servings: 6
Preparation time: 15 minutes
Cook time: 30 minutes
Ready in: 45 minutes

Nutrition Facts

Serving Size 123 g

Amount Per Serving

Calories 260   Calories from Fat 228

	% Daily Value*
Total Fat 25.4g	**39%**
Saturated Fat 14.9g	**74%**
Trans Fat 0.0g	
Cholesterol 123mg	**41%**
Sodium 177mg	**7%**
Total Carbohydrates 9.5g	**3%**
Dietary Fiber 1.0g	**4%**
Sugars 3.4g	
Protein 3.3g	

Vitamin A 17%	•	Vitamin C 62%
Calcium 4%	•	Iron 3%

Nutrition Grade D
* Based on a 2000 calorie diet

Ingredients
- 12 ounces strawberries
- 1/2 cup stevia
- 1/2 cup butter, softened
- 2 eggs
- 1/2 cup almond flour
- 1 teaspoon pure vanilla extract
- 1 pinch sea salt
- 1 cup heavy cream, whipped
- coconut oil for greasing

Directions
1. **Preheat** oven to 375 degrees F.
2. **Mix** strawberries with 1/4 cup stevia. Place fruit mixture in a 6x8 inch baking dish greased with coconut oil.

151

3. **Beat** butter and the remaining stevia until creamy. Add eggs and beat until curd-like texture. Beat in the almond flour and vanilla.
4. **Spoon** mixture over fruit and spread gradually.
5. **Bake** for 30 minutes or until topping is golden brown.
6. **Cool** slightly and top with whipped cream to serve.

9. Low Carb Zucchini Muffins

Servings: 12
Preparation time: 15 minutes
Cook time: 30 minutes
Ready in: 45 minutes

Nutrition Facts

Serving Size 164 g

Amount Per Serving

Calories 325   Calories from Fat 268

	% Daily Value*
Total Fat 29.8g	**46%**
Saturated Fat 7.5g	**37%**
Trans Fat 0.0g	
Cholesterol 51mg	**17%**
Sodium 33mg	**1%**
Total Carbohydrates 12.5g	**4%**
Dietary Fiber 4.5g	**18%**
Sugars 1.5g	
Protein 10.8g	

Vitamin A 4%	•	Vitamin C 2%
Calcium 11%	•	Iron 10%

Nutrition Grade D
* Based on a 2000 calorie diet

Ingredients
- 3 eggs, beaten
- 2 teaspoons pure vanilla extract
- 3/4 cup heavy cream
- 50g stevia
- 1/4 cup coconut oil, plus extra amount for greasing
- 1 1/4 teaspoons baking soda
- 1/8 teaspoon sea salt
- 3/4 cup grated zucchini, and squeezed
- 3 tablespoons wheat bran

- 3 1/2 cups almond flour
- 1/2 teaspoon ground cinnamon
- 1/2 teaspoon ground nutmeg
- 1 cup chopped walnuts

Directions

1. **Preheat** oven to 375 degrees F. Grease a 12-cup muffin tin with coconut oil.
2. **Beat** together the eggs, vanilla, heavy cream, and stevia. Add the coconut oil, baking soda, and salt, and stir to combine. Fold in the grated zucchini.
3. **Combine** wheat bran, almond flour, cinnamon, and nutmeg. Pour almond flour mixture into the zucchini mixture. Fold in chopped walnut then scoop batter among muffin cups.
4. **Bake** for 30 minutes, or until a toothpick inserted into the center comes out clean. Let it cool for a few minutes and serve.

10. Date Chocolate Truffles

Servings: 18
Ready in: 40 minutes

Nutrition Facts

Serving Size 25 g

Amount Per Serving

Calories 116   Calories from Fat 83

% Daily Value*

Total Fat 9.3g	**14%**
Saturated Fat 5.1g	**26%**
Cholesterol 0mg	**0%**
Sodium 29mg	**1%**
Total Carbohydrates 9.1g	**3%**
Dietary Fiber 2.0g	**8%**
Sugars 6.2g	
Protein 2.0g	

Vitamin A 0%	•	Vitamin C 1%
Calcium 1%	•	Iron 8%

Nutrition Grade C-
* Based on a 2000 calorie diet

Ingredients

- 20 dates, pitted
- 1 cup coconut flakes
- 3/4 cup toasted walnuts
- 1/4 cup coconut oil
- 2 ounces unsweetened chocolate, finely chopped
- 1 teaspoon pure vanilla extract
- 1/4 teaspoon sea salt

Directions

1. **Combine** dates, coconut flakes, walnuts, and coconut oil in a food processor. Process until finely ground.
2. **Melt** chocolate in a warm pan. Spoon the melted chocolate into the processor and add salt and vanilla. Process until well mixed.
3. **Transfer** mixture into a bowl and refrigerate for 30 minutes.
4. **Roll** mixture into balls and place on container and return it in the refrigerator until completely hardened. Keep cool until serving.

Books by Maggie Fitzgerald

The 7-Day Acid Reflux Diet

The 3-Step Diabetic Diet Plan

The Anti-Inflammatory Diet Plan

Ketogenic Diet Crash Course

Atkins Diet Beginners' Crash Course

www.amazon.com/author/robertfleischer

About Robert M. Fleischer

Besides being a noted author, Robert M. Fleischer is a California-based health researcher, husband and a father of 2 children, one boy and one girl. He has dedicated his career to developing better standards of care and treatment for patients of common, chronic and misunderstood conditions which are often handled with pharmaceuticals to treat the symptoms rather than lifestyle changes which address the root cause.

In his spare time he enjoys tennis, mountain biking and is a member of a local amateur theater group.

Exclusive Bonus Download: Healthy Chemistry for Optimal Health

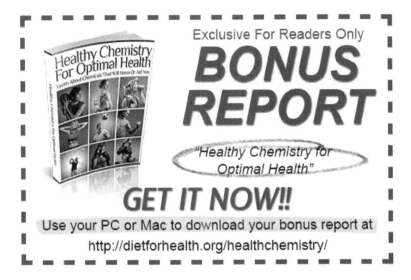

Download your bonus, please visit the download link above from your PC or MAC. To open PDF files, visit http://get.adobe.com/reader/ to download the reader if it's not already installed on your PC or Mac. To open ZIP files, you may need to download WinZip from http://www.winzip.com. This download is for PC or Mac ONLY and might not be downloadable to kindle.

Thousands Have Used Chemicals To Improve Their Medical Condition!

Is the fact that you would like to learn to use chemicals for your health but just don't know how and this is making your life difficult... maybe even miserable?

First, you are NOT alone! It may seem like it sometimes, but not knowing how to get better your skills is far more common than you'd think.

Your lack of knowledge in this area may not be your fault, but that doesn't mean that you shouldn't -- or can't -- do anything to find out everything you need to know to finally be a success!

So today -- in the next FEW MINUTES, in fact -- we're going to help you GET ON TRACK, and learn how you can quickly and easily get your skills under control... for GOOD!

With this product, and it's great information on chemicals it will walk you, each and every chemicals and it's use to help you get all the info you need to be health.

In This Book, You Will Learn:

- The Chemistry Of The Blood
- The Relationship Between The Biology And The Chemistry Of The Blood
- Dangerous Chemicals To The Body
- Good Chemicals To The Body
- 10 Reasons Why You Should Avoid The Bad Chemicals

And so much more!

Visit the URL above to download this guide and start improving your health NOW

One Last Thing...

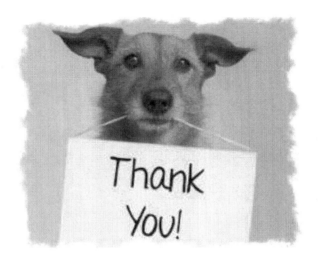

Thank you so much for reading my book. I hope you really liked it. As you probably know, many people look at the reviews on Amazon before they decide to purchase a book. If you liked the book, could you please take a minute to leave a review with your feedback? 60 seconds is all I'm asking for, and it would mean the world to me.

Robert M. Fleischer

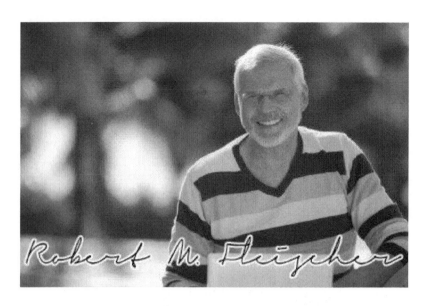

NaturalWay

Publishing

Atlanta, Georgia USA

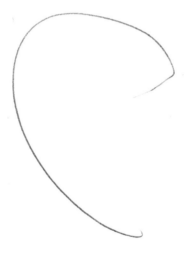

Made in the USA
Lexington, KY
16 April 2016